Study Guide to Accompany

Essentials of
Nursing Research

METHODS, APPRAISAL, AND UTILIZATION

FIFTH EDITION

D1491273

Denise F. Polit, PhD

President
Humanalysis, Inc.
Saratoga Springs, New York

Cheryl Tatano Beck, DNSc, CNM, FAAN

Professor
University of Connecticut, School of Nursing
Storrs, Connecticut

Bernadette P. Hungler, BSN, PhD

Visiting Lecturer
Regis College
Weston, Massachusetts

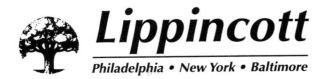

Lippincott

Philadelphia • New York • Baltimore

Study Guide to Accompany

Essentials of Nursing Research
METHODS, APPRAISAL, AND UTILIZATION

FIFTH EDITION

Ancillary Editor: *Doris S. Wray*
Senior Project Editor: *Erika Kors*
Senior Production Manager: *Helen Ewan*
Senior Production Coordinator: *Nannette Winski*

Fifth Edition

9 8 7 6 5 4 3 2

ISBN: 0–7817–2558–5

Care has been taken to confirm the accuracy of the information presented and to describe generally accepted practices. However, the authors, editors, and publisher are not responsible for errors or omissions or for any consequences from application of the information in this book and make no warranty, express or implied, with respect to the contents of the publication.

The authors, editors and publisher have exerted every effort to ensure that drug selection and dosage set forth in this text are in accordance with current recommendations and practice at the time of publication. However, in view of ongoing research, changes in government regulations, and the constant flow of information relating to drug therapy and drug reactions, the reader is urged to check the package insert for each drug for any change in indications and dosage and for added warnings and precautions. This is particularly important when the recommended agent is a new or infrequently employed drug.

Some drugs and medical devices presented in this publication have Food and Drug Administration (FDA) clearance for limited use in restricted research settings. It is the responsibility of the health care provider to ascertain the FDA status of each drug or device planned for use in their clinical practice.

Preface

This Study Guide has been prepared to complement the fifth edition of *Essentials of Nursing Research: Methods, Appraisal, and Utilization.* The guide provides opportunities to reinforce the acquisition of basic research skills through systematic learning exercises. The book is also intended to help bridge the gap between the passive reading of complex, abstract materials and active participation in the development of skills needed to evaluate research through concrete examples and study suggestions.

As in the case of the textbook, this Study Guide was developed on the premise that research examples are a critical component of the learning process. The inclusion of actual and fictitious research examples is designed to instruct (i.e., enhance the retention of research concepts), motivate (i.e., encourage you to appreciate the utility of acquiring research skills), and stimulate (i.e., suggest topics that you might well pursue as you think about utilizing research findings).

The Study Guide consists of sixteen chapters—one chapter corresponding to each chapter in the textbook. Each of the sixteen chapters (with a few exceptions) consists of five sections:

- *Matching Exercises.* Terms and concepts presented in the textbook are reinforced by having you perform a matching routine that often involves matching the concrete (e.g., actual hypotheses) with the abstract (e.g., type of hypotheses).
- *Completion Exercises.* Sentences are presented in which you must fill in a missing word or phrase corresponding to important ideas presented in the textbook.
- *Study Questions.* Each chapter contains two to five short individual exercises relevant to the materials in the textbook, including the preparation of definitions of terms.
- *Application Exercises.* These exercises are geared specifically to the consumers of nursing research and involve opportunities to critique various aspects of a study. Each chapter contains both fictitious research examples and suggestions for one or more actual research examples, which you are asked to evaluate according to a dimension emphasized in the corresponding chapter of the textbook.
- *Special Projects.* This section offers suggestions for fairly large projects in which, in many cases, an entire classroom could collaborate.

This Study Guide also includes two complete studies for your critical appraisal, supplementing the two complete studies included in the textbook.

The Appendix to this edition includes answers to selected Study Guide exercises so that you can get instant feedback on your progress. Finally, new to this edition is a self-study guide on a CD-ROM that contains over 200 multiple choice questions that allows you to review the content presented in the textbook. In Study Mode, you respond to the questions and get instant feedback, with the rationale for correct and incorrect answers. In Test Mode, you can take practice tests covering individual chapters or clusters of chapters; the practice tests are scored, and feedback is available for your review at the conclusion.

Contents

PART VI
Critical Appraisal and Utilization of Nursing Research

PART VII
Research Reports

PART I

Overview of Nursing Research

CHAPTER 1

Exploring Nursing Research

■ A. Matching Exercises

1. Match each of the activities in Set B with one of the timeframes in Set A. Indicate the letter corresponding to the appropriate response next to each entry in Set B.

SET A

a. Pre-1970s

b. 1970s and 1980s

c. 1990s to present

d. None of the above

SET B   **RESPONSES**

1. Nursing research focused on nurses themselves. _____

2. Shift in research focus to clinical problems. _____

3. Establishment of the National Institute of Nursing Research at the National Institutes of Health. _____

4. Conferences on Research Priorities (CORP) are convened. _____

5. Issue of research utilization becomes more prominent. _____

6. Creation of the professional journal *Nursing Research*. _____

7. Increased focus on outcomes research. _____

8. Federal funding becomes available to support nursing research. _____

9. Greater interest in qualitative research, as evidenced by creation of the journal *Qualitative Health Research*. _____

10. Two professional nursing research journals cease publication due to low circulation. _____

2. Match each statement in Set B with one of the paradigms in Set A. Indicate the letter corresponding to the appropriate response next to each entry in Set B.

SET A

a. Positivist paradigm

b. Naturalist paradigm

c. Neither paradigm

d. Both paradigms

SET B   RESPONSES

1. Assumes that reality exists and that it can be objectively
   studied and known.   _____

2. Subjectivity in inquiries is considered inevitable
   and desirable.   _____

3. Inquiries rely on external, empirical evidence that is
   collected through human senses.   _____

4. Develops knowledge primarily through deductive
   processes.   _____

5. Assumes reality is a construction and that many
   constructions are possible.   _____

6. Relies primarily on the collection and analysis of
   quantitative information.   _____

7. Relies primarily on the collection and analysis of
   narrative, qualitative information.   _____

8. Provides a framework for inquiries undertaken by
   nurse researchers.   _____

9. Inquiries give rise to emerging interpretations that are
   grounded in people's experiences.   _____

10. Inquiries are not constrained by ethical issues.   _____

11. Has its roots in nineteenth-century philosophers such
    as Comte, Mill, Newton, and Locke.   _____

12. Inquiries focus on discrete, specific concepts while
    attempting to control other aspects of a phenomenon.   _____

■ B. Completion Exercises

Write the words or phrases that correctly complete the sentences below.

1. Research in nursing began with _____.

2. During the early years, most nursing studies focused on _____
   _____.

3. The future direction of nursing research is likely to involve a continuing focus on _____.

4. The most ingrained source of knowledge, and the one that is the most difficult to challenge, is _____.

5. The process of developing generalizations from specific observations is referred to as _____ reasoning.

6. The scientific approach has as its philosophical underpinnings a school of thought known as _____.

7. The assumption that all phenomena have antecedent causes is called _____.

8. The _____ paradigm is sometimes referred to as the phenomenologic or constructivist paradigm.

9. The approach to human knowledge that uses systematic, controlled procedures is known as the _____.

10. Evidence that is rooted in objective reality and gathered through the human senses is known as _____ evidence.

11. Because scientific inquiry is not concerned with isolated phenomena, a key characteristic of the scientific method is _____.

12. Researchers who reject the classical model of scientific inquiry criticize it for being overly _____.

13. Naturalistic inquiry always takes place in the _____ _____, in naturalistic settings.

14. The type of research that involves the systematic collection and analysis of controlled, numerical information is known as _____.

15. The type of research that involves the systematic collection and analysis of subjective, narrative materials is known as _____.

16. A specific aim of some qualitative research that asks "What is the name of this phenomenon?" is referred to as _____.

■ C. Study Questions

1. Define the following terms. Compare your definition with the definition in Chapter 1 or in the glossary.

a. Evidence-based practice _____
_____.

b. Producer of nursing research _____
_____.

c. Consumer of nursing research _____
_____.

d. National Institute of Nursing Research _____
_____.

e. Outcomes research _____
_____.

f. Replication _____
_____.

g. Deductive reasoning _____
_____.

h. Inductive reasoning _____
_____.

i. Assumption _____
_____.

j. Paradigm _____
_____.

k. Logical positivism _____
_____.

l. Naturalistic paradigm _____
_____.

m. Scientific method _____
_____.

n. Empiricism _____
_____.

o. Applied research _____
_____.

p. Basic research _____

_____.

2. Why is it important for nurses who will never conduct their own research to understand scientific methods?

_____

_____

_____

_____

_____

3. What are some potential consequences to the profession of nursing if nurses stopped conducting their own research?

_____

_____

_____

_____

_____

4. Students sometimes have concerns about courses on research methods. Complete the following sentences, expressing as honestly as possible your own feelings about research, and discuss your concerns with your class.

   a. I (am/am not) looking forward to this class on nursing research because:

   _____

   _____

   b. I think that I would like a course in nursing research methods better if:

   _____

   _____

   c. I think that a class in nursing research (will/will not) improve my effectiveness as a nurse because:

   _____

   _____

5. Below are several research problems. For each, indicate whether you think it is *primarily* an applied or basic research question. Justify your response.

a. Does movement tempo affect perception of the passage of time?

_____

_____

b. Does follow-up by nurses improve patients' compliance with their medication regimens?

_____

_____

c. Does the ingestion of cranberry juice reduce urinary tract infections?

_____

_____

d. Is sweat gland activity related to ACTH levels?

_____

_____

e. Is pain perception associated with a person's locus of control (an aspect of personality)?

_____

_____

f. Does the type of nursing curriculum affect attrition rates in schools of nursing?

_____

_____

g. Does nicotine affect postural muscle tremor?

_____

_____

h. Does the nurse/patient ratio affect nurses' job satisfaction?

_____

_____

6. Below are descriptions of several research problems. Indicate whether you think the problem is best suited to a qualitative or quantitative approach and indicate why you think this is so.

a. What is the decision-making process of AIDS patients seeking treatment?

_____

_____

b. What effect does room temperature have on the colonization rate of bacteria in urinary catheters?

_____

_____

c. What are the sources of stress among nursing home residents?

_____

_____

d. Does therapeutic touch affect the vital signs of hospitalized patients?

_____

_____

e. What is the process by which nursing students acquire a professional nursing identity?

_____

_____

f. What are the effects of prenatal instruction on the labor and delivery outcomes of pregnant women?

_____

_____

g. What are the health care needs of the homeless, and what are the barriers they face in having those needs met?

_____

_____

7. What are some of the limitations of quantitative research? What are some of the limitations of qualitative research? Which approach seems best suited to address problems in which you might be interested? Why is that?

_____

_____

_____

_____

_____

■ D. Application Exercises

1. Below is a brief description of a fictitious study, followed by a critique. Do you agree with the critique? Can you add other comments relevant to issues discussed in Chapter 1 of the textbook? (Box 1-1 offers some guiding questions.)

Fictitious Study. Singleton (2001) studied a sample of 100 nurses to determine whether the setting in which they practiced was related to their attitudes toward caring for patients with acquired immunodeficiency syndrome (AIDS). The settings chosen were acute hospital, hospice home care, clinics, and long-term care facilities. Each nurse completed a paper-and-pencil questionnaire comprised of 20 questions. The questions asked them to rate (on a scale from 1 to 10) how important they considered physical care, help in dying, hope, protection of themselves, and other aspects of caring for AIDS patients. The researchers found that a higher percentage of nurses employed by acute care facilities believed that physical care and hope were important in caring for people with AIDS than did nurses employed in other settings. Nurses in all four types of settings identified protection of self as the most important aspect of care.

Critique. Although this study focused on a topic that is of great current interest, its relevance to nursing practice seems indirect. The researchers studied nurses' attitudes toward caring rather than focusing on actual nursing care. Studies examining problems encountered in the delivery of care, methods for helping patients with AIDS cope with the disease and death, or the timing of ministrations to reduce nausea or enhance nourishment would have been considerably more relevant to the practice of nursing. Studies focusing on people with AIDS are needed because of the ever-increasing number of people with the diagnosis. They represent a group with special needs and are a high-priority group for research inquiry. Redirecting the focus of the study to nursing care or to the needs of victims of this critical health problem would make it more useful. This brief abstract does not provide much information about the researcher's purpose and methodologic approach; however, it appears that Singleton's study was quantitative (for instance, she was able to compute percentages). The study described nurses' attitudes and explored the relation between attitudes and type of practice setting. The study generated some basic information about nurses' attitudes, but presumably the researcher intended to apply this knowledge in some fashion (e.g., to identify needs for training or education or to use the findings as a basis for discussions among nurses about caring for patients with AIDS).

2. Below is a summary of a fictitious study. Read the summary and then respond to the questions that follow.

Nicolet (2000) studied the effect of the wording of communications on encouraging the elderly to come forward for a flu vaccination. All members of a senior citizens' center in a middle-sized community (a total of 500 elderly men and women) were sent a letter advising them that a flu epidemic was anticipated and that the elderly were especially likely to benefit from an immunization. Half of the members were sent a letter stressing the benefits of getting a flu shot. The other half of the members were sent a letter stressing the potential dangers of *not* getting a flu shot. To avoid any biases, a lottery-type system was used to determine who got which letter. All the elderly were advised that free immunizations would be available at a community health clinic over a one-week period and that free transportation would also be made available to them. Nicolet monitored the rates of coming forward for a flu shot among the two groups of elderly to assess whether one approach of encouragement was more persuasive than the other.

Consider the aspects of this study in relationship to the issues discussed in this chapter. To assist you in your review, here are some guiding questions:

a. Discuss the relevance of this study to nursing.

b. Do the methods used in this study suggest that the underlying paradigm is positivism or naturalism? Would it be more appropriate to collect and analyze qualitative or quantitative information? Why do you think this is so?

c. How would you characterize the purpose of this study? Is its major aim identification, description, exploration, explanation, prediction, or control? Is there more than one purpose?

d. Would you say this study is an example of basic or applied research?

3. A second brief summary of a fictitious study follows. Read the summary and then respond to questions **a** to **d** from Question D.2 in terms of this study.

Ryan (2000) designed a study to explore and describe the meaning of the risk experience among middle-aged men and women whose parents had died of colon cancer and who, therefore, were at elevated risk for colon cancer themselves. A sample of 15 people whose parents had died within the previous twelve months were recruited for the study. In-depth interviews, lasting between one and two hours, were conducted in the sample members' homes. The interviews were tape-recorded and later transcribed. The interviews examined such issues as perceptions of risk, factors contributing to the perceptions, stress associated with risk perceptions, risk reduction efforts, and coping strategies.

4. Below are several suggested research articles. Skim one or more of these articles and respond to parts **a** to **d** of Question D.2 in terms of an actual research study.

- Corbett, C. A., & Callister, L. C. (2000). Nursing support during labor. *Clinical Nursing Research, 9,* 70–83.
- Hutchinson, M. K. (1998). Something to talk about: Sexual risk communication between young women and their partners. *Journal of Obstetric, Gynecologic, and Neonatal Nursing, 27,* 127–133.
- Jacobs, V. (2000). Informational needs of surgical patients following discharge. *Applied Nursing Research, 13,* 12–18.
- McDonald, D. D. (1999). Postoperative pain after hospital discharge. *Clinical Nursing Research, 8,* 355–367.
- Warda, M. R. (2000). Mexican Americans' perceptions of culturally competent care. *Western Journal of Nursing Research, 22,* 203–224.

■ E. Special Projects

1. Consider the following research statement:

   The purpose of this study is to determine whether patients in intensive care units are or are not satisfied with their nursing care.

   The basic purpose of this study as stated is descriptive. Alter the statement in such a way as to design a study whose essential purpose is exploration; explanation; prediction; and control.

2. Think of the last "fact" you learned with respect to clinical nursing practice. Try to discover the ultimate source of this information. Was it tradition ("This is the way it's always been done")? Authority ("Dr. So-and-so said so")? Logical reasoning ("This has been inferred from previous observations")? Or systematic research ("An empirical investigation discovered this to be the case")?

CHAPTER 2

Comprehending the Research Process

■ A. Matching Exercises

1. Match each of the terms in Set B with one of the responses in Set A. Indicate the letter corresponding to your response next to each item in Set B.

SET A

a. Term used in quantitative research
b. Term used in qualitative research
c. Term used in both qualitative or quantitative research

SET B   **RESPONSES**

1. Subject   _____

2. Study participant   _____

3. Informant   _____

4. Variable   _____

5. Phenomena   _____

6. Construct   _____

7. Theory   _____

8. Data   _____

2. Match each of the terms in Set B with one (or more) of the terms in Set A. Indicate the letter(s) corresponding to your response next to each item in Set B.

SET A

a. Categorical variable
b. Continuous variable
c. Constant

SET B   RESPONSES

1. Employment status (working/not working).   _____

2. Dosage of a new drug.   _____

3. Pi (π) (to calculate area of a circle).   _____

4. Number of aspirins consumed annually.   _____

5. Method of teaching patients (structured versus
   unstructured).   _____

6. Blood type.   _____

7. pH level of urine.   _____

8. Pulse rate of a deceased person.   _____

9. Membership (versus nonmembership) in a nursing
   organization.   _____

10. Birth weight of an infant.   _____

11. Presence or absence of decubitus.   _____

12. Body temperature.   _____

3. Match each of the terms in Set B with one of the terms in Set A. Indicate
   the letter corresponding to your response next to each item in Set B.

SET A

a. Independent variable

b. Dependent variable

c. Either/both

SET B   RESPONSES

1. The variable that is the presumed effect   _____

2. The variable that is dichotomous   _____

3. The variable that is the main outcome of interest in the study   _____

4. The variable that is the presumed cause   _____

5. The variable that is continuous   _____

6. The variable that is an attribute   _____

7. The variable, "length of stay in hospital"   _____

8. The variable that requires an operational definition   _____

■ B. Completion Exercises

Write the words or phrases that correctly complete the sentences below.

1. The person who undertakes a research project is known as the
   _____ or _____.

2. In a quantitative study, the people who are being studied in a research
   project are often referred to as the _____,
   but they may be referred to as the _____
   in both qualitative and quantitative studies.

3. The abstract qualities that a researcher is interested in are referred to by
   both qualitative and quantitative researchers as _____
   _____.

4. A _____, a term used primarily in quanti-
   tative research, is a quality of a person, group, setting, or situation that
   takes on different values.

5. A _____ variable is one that takes on only
   a few discrete values.

6. Whereas gender is a categorical variable, height is a(n) _____
   _____ variable.

7. The variable presumed to *cause* or influence changes in some other variable is the _____.

8. The variable that the researcher wants to understand, explain, or predict
   is known as the _____ variable.

9. If a researcher studied the effect of a scheduling assignment on nurses'
   morale, the scheduling assignment would be referred to as the _____
   _____ variable.

10. The pieces of information obtained in the course of a study are collec-
    tively known as the _____.

11. When a quantitative researcher carefully specifies the steps that must be
    taken to measure the concepts of interest, the researcher develops
    _____.

12. When the data are in the form of narrative descriptions, the data are said
    to be _____.

13. While quantitative researchers are often interested in studying relation-
    ships between variables, qualitative researchers examine _____
    _____.

14. "The higher the caloric intake, the greater the weight" expresses a presumed _____ relationship.

15. "Men are more likely to suffer depression following the death of their spouses than women" expresses a presumed _____ relationship.

16. When little is known about a topic or phenomenon, _____ research is likely to be more fruitful than _____ research.

17. There is typically a well-defined, prespecified set of activities with fairly linear progression in a _____ study.

18. The overall plan for collecting and analyzing research data is called the

    _____.

19. The actual group of people selected from a larger group to participate in a study is known as the _____.

20. Typically, the most time-consuming phase of the study is the

    _____ phase.

21. The task of organizing and synthesizing the information collected in a study is known as _____.

22. A small-scale trial run of a research study is referred to as a(n)

    _____.

23. The findings from an investigation are communicated in a

    _____.

24. The final phase of a research project is known as the _____ phase.

25. In a qualitative study, an important activity after identifying a research site is developing a strategy for _____ into selected settings within the site.

26. Quantitative researchers decide in advance how many study participants to include in a study, but qualitative researchers' sampling decisions are often guided by the principle of _____ of the data.

■ C. Study Questions

1. Define the following concepts. Compare your definitions with those in Chapter 2 or in the glossary.

    a. Informant _____

    _____

b. Subject _____

_____

c. Construct _____

_____

d. Variable _____

_____

e. Heterogeneity _____

_____

f. Categorical variable _____

_____

g. Operational definition _____

_____

h. Relationship _____

_____

i. Cause-and-effect relationship _____

_____

j. Functional relationship _____

_____

k. Research control _____

_____

l. Data collection plan _____

_____

m. Sampling plan _____

_____

n. Raw data _____

_____

2. Suggest operational definitions for the following concepts.

a. Stress _____

_____

b. Prematurity of infants _____

_____

c. Nursing effectiveness _____

_____

d. Knowledge of critical care nursing concepts _____

_____

e. Nurses' educational preparation _____

_____

f. Patient recovery _____

_____

g. Prolonged labor _____

_____

h. Smoking behavior _____

_____

i. Nurses' job dissatisfaction _____

_____

j. Respiratory function _____

_____

3. In each of the following research problems, identify the independent and dependent variables.

a. Does assertiveness training improve the effectiveness of psychiatric nurses?

Independent _____

Dependent _____

b. Does the postural positioning of patients affect their respiratory function?

Independent _____

Dependent _____

c. Is the psychological well-being of patients affected by the amount of touch received from nursing staff?

Independent _____

Dependent _____

d. Is the incidence of decubiti reduced by more frequent turnings of patients?

Independent _____

Dependent _____

e. Is the educational preparation of nurses related to their subsequent turnover rate?

Independent _____

Dependent _____

f. Is tolerance for pain related to a patient's age and gender?

Independent _____

Dependent _____

g. Are the number of prenatal visits of pregnant women associated with labor and delivery outcomes?

Independent _____

Dependent _____

h. Are levels of stress among nurses higher in pediatric or adult intensive care units?

Independent _____

Dependent _____

i. Are nursing students' clinical grades related to their subsequent on-the-job performances?

Independent _____

Dependent _____

j. Is anxiety in surgical patients affected by structured preoperative teaching?

Independent _____

Dependent _____

k. Are nurses' promotions related to their level of participation in continuing education activities?

Independent _____

Dependent _____

l. Does hearing acuity of the elderly change as a function of the time of day?

Independent _____

Dependent _____

m. Is patient satisfaction with nursing care related to the congruity of nurses' and patients' cultural backgrounds?

Independent _____

Dependent _____

n. Is a woman's educational attainment related to the frequency of breast self-examination?

Independent _____

Dependent _____

o. Does home birth affect the parents' satisfaction with the childbirth experience?

Independent _____

Dependent _____

■ D. Application Exercises

1. Below is a brief description of certain aspects of a fictitious study, followed by a critique. Do you agree with the critique? Can you add other comments relevant to issues discussed in Chapter 2 of the textbook? (Boxes 1-1 and 2-3 offer some guiding questions.)

Fictitious Study. Kettlewell (2001) studied factors affecting the duration of breastfeeding among low-income women living in an urban community. The factors under scrutiny were the mothers' educational attainment, their level of depression, and their race and ethnicity. The variables in the study were defined as follows:

- Breastfeeding duration: The age of the child (in weeks) when he or she was totally weaned from the breast.
- Educational attainment: The highest grade in school that the mother completed.
- Level of depression: The mother's score on the Center for Epidemiological Studies Depression (CES-D) Scale.
- Race and ethnicity: Whether the mother was African American, white, or Hispanic.

Critique. There are four concepts (variables) in Kettlewell's study. The dependent variable is breastfeeding duration, and the independent variables are educational attainment, level of depression, and race and ethnicity. Kettlewell is interested in knowing whether a mother's decision to prolong or curtail breastfeeding is related to how far she went in school, how depressed she is, and what her cultural background is.

Although we do not have much information about the design of Kettlewell's study, we do know that she controlled at least two variables: socioeconomic status and area of residence. The study focused exclusively on low-income urban women; thus, income and urban residence were, in this study, not allowed to vary. Holding these variables constant enhanced Kettlewell's ability to interpret the results of her study.

Kettlewell's operational definitions appear to be reasonably good, but they could be expanded to indicate how the data would be collected. For example, for the dependent variable (breastfeeding duration), the definition might be the age of the child (in weeks) when he or she was totally weaned from the breast, as reported by the mother in an interview completed when the child was 2 years old.

2. Below is a summary of a fictitious study. Read the summary and then respond to the questions that follow.

Portnoy and Stamm (2000) observed that different patients react differently to sensory overload in the hospital. They conducted a study to see whether the patients' home environments affect their reactions to hospital noises. Below are the investigators' operational definitions of the research variables.

Independent Variable: Type of home environment. Based on the patients' self-reports at intake, home environment was defined as the number of household members residing with the patient.

Dependent Variable: Reaction to hospital noise. Based on responses to five questions (agree/disagree type) answered at discharge, patients were classified as "dissatisfied with noise level" or "not dissatisfied with noise level."

Other Variables

Age: Calculated to the nearest year based on birth date reported at intake

Gender: Patient's gender as recorded on intake form

Social class: Patient's occupation as recorded on intake form

Review and comment on these specifications. Suggest alternatives and compare the adequacy and completeness of your suggestions with the descriptions provided above. To aid you in this task, here are some guiding questions:

a. Identify which variables in this study were categorical, discrete, and continuous.

b. Are the operational definitions of the research variables sufficiently detailed? Do they tell the reader exactly how each variable is to be measured? Can you expand any of the definitions so that they are more precise?

c. Are the operational definitions good definitions—that is, is there a better way to measure the research variables?

d. What type of relationship is implied by the research question—a functional or causal relationship?

e. This study is quantitative—is the question the researchers posed appropriate for a quantitative inquiry? Would a more qualitatively oriented approach have been more appropriate?

3. Below are several suggested research articles for quantitative studies. Read one of these articles and identify the independent variable(s) and dependent variable(s) of the study. Also, respond to questions a through e from Question D.2 with regard to this actual research study.

■ Anderson, M. A., Helms, L. B., Black, S., & Myers, D. K. (2000). A rural perspective on home care communication about elderly patients after hospital discharge. *Western Journal of Nursing Research, 22,* 225–243.

■ Greif, J., Hewitt, W., & Armstrong, M. L. (2000). Tattooing and body piercing: Body art practices among college students. *Clinical Nursing Research, 8,* 368–385.

■ Lauri, S. et al. (1998). Decision making of nurses practicing in intensive care in Canada, Finland, Northern Ireland, Switzerland, and the United States. *Heart & Lung, 27,* 133–142.

■ Sittner, B., Hudson, D. B., Grossman, C. C., & Gaston-Johansson, F. (1998). Adolescents' perceptions of pain during labor. *Clinical Nursing Research, 7,* 82–93.

■ Souder, E., & O'Sullivan, P. S. (2000). Nursing documentation versus standardized assessment of cognitive status is hospitalized medical patients. *Applied Nursing Research, 13,* 29–36.

4. A second brief description of a fictitious study follows. Read the description and then respond to the questions that follow.

Godine and Nicholson (2000) undertook a study to understand the meaning of compliance with a medical regimen from the patient's perspective among low-income rural patients with chronic health problems. Godine and Nicholson noted that although compliance is a widely researched phenomenon, the patient's viewpoint is often ignored. The researchers recruited a sample of 18 men and women ranging in age from 27 to 68 from a health clinic in rural Tennessee. The in-depth interviews, which lasted about 90 minutes on average, were conducted at the clinic. The interviews focused on the nature of the chronic health problem, the nature of the therapeutic regimen, and the meaning of compliance from the informants' perspectives.

Review and comment on this study. To aid you in this task, here are some guiding questions:
   a. What is the central phenomenon under study in this research project?
   b. Is the question the researchers posed appropriate for a qualitative inquiry? Would a more quantitatively oriented approach have been more appropriate?
   c. What types of patterns of association, if any, were explored?
   d. What is the setting for the study? Was this setting appropriate? How difficult do you think it was to gain entrée into this setting?

5. Below are several suggested research articles for qualitative studies. Read one of these articles and respond to parts **a** to **d** of Question D.4 in critiquing this actual research study.

■ Beck, C. T. (1996). Postpartum depressed mothers' experiences interacting with their children. *Nursing Research, 45,* 98–109.

■ Chiu, L. (2000). Lived experience of spirituality in Taiwanese women with breast cancer. *Western Journal of Nursing Research, 22,* 29–53.

■ Kee, C. C. (1998). Living with osteoarthritis: Insiders' view. *Applied Nursing Research, 11,* 19–26.

■ Volume, C. I. (2000). Hoping to maintain a balance: The concept of hope and the discontinuation of anorexiant medications. *Qualitative Health Research, 10,* 174–187.

■ E. Special Projects

1. Suppose you were interested in studying the effect of a hysterectomy on women's sexuality and sexual identity. Briefly outline what you might do in the following tasks, as outlined in this chapter:

   Step 4: Formulate hypotheses

   Step 5: Select a research design

   Step 6: Identify the population

   Step 7: Specify the methods to measure or operationalize the variables

   Step 8: Select a sample

2. Think of five pairs of variables that might have a relationship between them (e.g., smoking status and lung cancer status). For each pair, indicate whether you presume the relationship to be functional or causal.

3. Suppose that a researcher wanted to do a qualitative study of a couple's decision to seek treatment for infertility. What types of sites and settings might be appropriate for such a study? Describe some steps the researcher might have to take to gain entrée into appropriate research settings.

CHAPTER 3

Reading Research Reports

■ A. Matching Exercises

1. Match each statement from Part B with one of the sections in a research report, as listed in Set A. Indicate the letter corresponding to your response next to each of the statements in Set B.

SET A

a. Abstract
b. Introduction
c. Method
d. Results
e. Discussion

SET B   **RESPONSES**

1. Describes the research design.   _____

2. In quantitative studies, presents the statistical analyses.   _____

3. Identifies the research questions or hypotheses.   _____

4. Presents a brief summary of the major features of the study.   _____

5. Provides information on study participants and how they
   were selected.   _____

6. Offers an interpretation of the study findings.   _____

7. In qualitative studies, describes the themes that emerged
   from the data.   _____

8. Offers a rationale for the study and describes its significance.   _____

9. Describes how the research data were collected.   _____

10. Identifies the study's main limitations.   _____

11. This sentence would appear there: "The purpose
    of this study is to explore the process by which patients
    cope with a cancer diagnosis."   _____

12. Includes raw data, in the form of excerpts, in qualitative reports.

_____

■ B. Completion Exercises

Write the words or phrases that correctly complete the sentences below.

1. Research findings summarized at a professional conference can be presented in one of two formats: _____ or _____.

2. The type of research reports that students are most likely to read are _____.

3. The _____ of a research report succinctly conveys the nature of the study to prospective readers.

4. Traditional abstracts are a single summary paragraph, but the newer-style abstracts are somewhat longer and have specific _____.

5. In a qualitative research report, the _____ would describe the central phenomenon under study.

6. "The data were collected by conducting face-to-face interviews with a sample of 100 nursing home residents" is a sentence most likely to appear in the _____ section of a research report.

7. A _____ is a procedure used in quantitative studies for testing hypotheses and evaluating the believability of the results.

8. In statistical testing, the _____ indicates how probable it is that the findings are reliable.

9. In a qualitative report, results are often organized according to major _____.

10. The following sentence would most likely appear in the _____ section of a research report: "These findings suggest that women who are physically abused are more likely to suffer from depression and fatigue than nonabused women."

■ C. Study Questions

1. Define the following terms. Compare your definitions with those in Chapter 3 or in the glossary.

a. Peer reviewer _____

_____

b. "Blind" review _____

_____

c. Poster session _____

_____

d. Research findings _____

_____

e. Statistical significance _____

_____

f. Research critique _____

_____

2. Why are qualitative research reports generally easier to read than quantitative research reports?

_____

_____

_____

_____

_____

3. Read one of the following articles and rewrite its abstract as a "new style" abstract with specific subheadings:

a. Christopher, K. A. (2000). Determinants of psychological well-being in Irish immigrants. *Western Journal of Nursing Research, 22,* 123–143.
b. Li, H., Stewart, B. J., Imle, M. A., Archbold, P. G., & Felver, L. (2000). Families and hospitalized elders: A typology of family care actions. *Research in Nursing & Health, 23,* 3–16.
c. Taylor, E. J., Highfield, M. F., & Amenta, M. (1999). Predictors of oncology and hospice nurses' spiritual care perspectives and practices. *Applied Nursing Research, 12,* 30–37.

4. Read the titles of the journal articles appearing in the February 2000 issue of *Applied Nursing Research* (or some other issue of this journal). Evaluate the titles of the articles in terms of length and adequacy in communicating essential information about the studies.

■ D. Application Exercises

1. Below is a brief abstract of a fictitious study, followed by a critique. Do you agree with the critique? Can you add other comments relevant to issues discussed in Chapter 3 of the textbook?

Fictitious Study. Forester (2000) prepared the following abstract for her study:

> Family members often experience considerable anxiety while their loved ones are in surgery. This study examined the effectiveness of a nursing intervention that involved providing oral intraoperative progress reports to family members. Surgical patients undergoing elective procedures were selected to either have family members receive the intervention or to not have them receive it. The findings indicated that the family members in the intervention group were less anxious than family members who received the usual care.

Critique. This brief abstract provides a general overview of the nature of Forester's study. It indicates a rationale for the study (the high anxiety level of surgical patients' family members) and summarizes what the researcher did. However, the abstract could well have provided more information while still staying within a 200-word guideline (the abstract only contains 77 words). For example, the abstract could have better described the nature of the intervention (e.g., at what point during the operation was information given to family members? How much detail was provided? etc.). For a reader to have a preliminary assessment of the worth of the study—and therefore to make a decision about whether to read the entire report—more information about the methods would also have been helpful. For example, the abstract should have indicated such methodological features as how the researcher measured anxiety and how many surgical patients were in the sample. Some indication of the study's implications would also have enhanced the usefulness of the abstract.

2. Below is an abstract from a fictitious study by Kachidurian (2001). Read the abstract and then respond to the questions that follow.

The purpose of this study was to evaluate the effectiveness of water pillows in reducing bilateral head flattening in preterm infants. The sample consisted of 46 healthy infants who were 35 weeks or less gestational age. Half the subjects, at random, received the special intervention, which involved having their heads supported on a small water pillow. The other 23 infants received customary care. The dependent variable was infant head shape, assessed using cranial measurements indicative of the roundness or flatness of the head. The two groups of infants had significantly different head measurements: the heads of those in the treatment group maintained a round shape, while those of the other infants became flattened. The findings thus suggest that the use of a small water pillow can help to alleviate bilateral head flattening in preterm infants, although replication of this study is warranted.

    a. Was this abstract readily comprehensible, even to readers with limited experience reading research reports?

    b. Did the abstract answer the following questions:

       (1) What were the research questions?

       (2) What methods did the researcher use to address those questions?

       (3) What did the researcher discover?

       (4) What are the implications for nursing practice?

    c. Is there any additional information that would have helped readers better understand the main features of the study?

3. Read the abstract for one of the articles listed below. Critique the abstract, applying questions a through c from Question D.2 above.

■ Boydell, K. M., Goering, P., & Morrell-Bellai, T. L. (2000). Narratives of identity: Re-presentation of self in people who are homeless. *Qualitative Health Research, 10,* 26–38.

■ DeFloor, T. (2000). The effect of position and mattress on interface pressure. *Applied Nursing Research, 13,* 2–11.

■ Fuller, B. F., Neu, M., & Smith, M. (1999). The influence of background clinical data on infant pain assessments. *Clinical Nursing Research, 8,* 179–187.

■ Keller, M. L., vonSadovzky, C., Pankratz, B., & Hermsen, J. (2000). Self-disclosure of HPV infection to sexual partners. *Western Journal of Nursing Research, 22,* 285–302.

■ Li, S., Holm, K., Gulanick, M., & Lanuza, D. (2000). Perimenopause and the quality of life. *Clinical Nursing Research, 9,* 6–26.

■ E. Special Projects

1. Prepare a title for the study described in Application Exercise D.1.

2. Read one of the studies suggested in Question D.3. Write a two-page summary of the research report, "translating" the information into everyday (i.e., nonresearch) language.

CHAPTER 4

Understanding the Ethics of Nursing Research

■ A. Matching Exercises

1. Match each of the descriptions in Set B with one of the procedures used to safeguard human subjects listed in Set A. Indicate the letter corresponding to the appropriate response next to each entry in Set B.

SET A

a. Freedom from harm or exploitation

b. Informed consent

c. Anonymity

d. Confidentiality

SET B   **RESPONSES**

1. A questionnaire distributed by mail bears an identification number in one corner. Respondents are assured their responses will not be individually divulged.   _____

2. Hospitalized children included in a study, and their parents, are told the aims and procedures of the research. Parents are asked to sign an authorization.   _____

3. Respondents in a questionnaire study in which the same respondents will be questioned twice are asked to place their own four-digit identification number on the questionnaire and to memorize the number. Respondents are assured their answers will remain private.   _____

4. Study participants in an in-depth study of family members' coping with a natural disaster renegotiate the terms of their participation at successive interviews.   _____

5. Women who recently had mastectomies are studied in terms of psychological sequelae. In the interview, sensitive questions are carefully worded. After the interview, debriefing with the respondent determines the need for psychological support.   _____

SET B   **RESPONSES**

6. Women interviewed in the above study (question 5) are told
    that the information they provide will not be individually
    divulged.   _____

7. Subjects who volunteered for an experimental treatment
    for AIDS are warned of potential side effects and are asked
    to sign a waiver.   _____

8. After determining that a new intervention resulted in
    discomfort to subjects, the researcher discontinued the
    study.   _____

9. Unmarked questionnaires are distributed to a class of
    nursing students. The instructions indicate that the
    responses will not be individually divulged.   _____

10. The researcher assures subjects that they will be
    interviewed as part of the study at a single point in time
    and adheres to this promise.   _____

11. A questionnaire distributed to a sample of nursing students
    includes a statement indicating that completion and
    submission of the questionnaire will be construed as
    voluntary participation in a study, as fully described in
    an accompanying letter.   _____

12. The names, ages, and occupations of study participants
    whose interviews are excerpted in the research report are
    not divulged.   _____

■ B. Completion Exercises

Write the words or phrases that correctly complete the sentences below.

1. Ethical _____ arise when the rights of subjects
    and the demands of science are put into direct conflict.

2. One of the first internationally recognized efforts to establish ethical
    standards was the _____ .

3. The National Commission for the Protection of Human Subjects of Bio-
    medical and Behavioral Research issued a well-known set of guidelines
    known as the _____.

4. The most straightforward ethical precept is the protection of subjects
    from _____ .

5. Risks that are no greater than those ordinarily encountered in daily life are referred to as _____.

6. The right to _____ means that prospective subjects have the right to voluntarily decide whether to participate in a study, without risk of penalty.

7. The researcher adheres to the principle of _____ by fully describing to subjects the nature of the study and the likely risks and benefits of participation.

8. When the researcher cannot link research information to the person who provided it, the condition known as _____ has prevailed.

9. Special procedures are often required to safeguard the rights of _____ subjects.

10. Committees established in institutions to review proposed research procedures with respect to their adherence to ethical guidelines are often called IRBs, or _____.

■ C. Study Questions

1. Define the following terms. Compare your definitions with those in Chapter 4 of the textbook or in the glossary.

   a. Code of ethics _____

   _____

   b. Beneficence _____

   _____

   c. Debriefing _____

   _____

   d. Stipend _____

   _____

   e. Risk/benefit ratio _____

   _____

   f. Process consent _____

   _____

   g. Covert data collection _____

   _____

h. Confidentiality _____

_____

i. Informed consent _____

_____

j. Vulnerable subjects _____

_____

k. Implied consent _____

_____

2. Below are descriptions of several research studies. Suggest some ethical dilemmas that are likely to emerge for each.

   a. An in-depth study of coping behaviors among rape victims _____

   _____

   b. An unobtrusive observational study of fathers' behaviors in the delivery room _____

   _____

   c. An interview study of the antecedents of heroin addiction _____

   _____

   d. A study of dependence among mentally retarded children _____

   _____

   e. An investigation of the verbal interactions among schizophrenic patients _____

   _____

   f. A study of the effects of a new drug on humans _____

   _____

3. The following two studies involved the use of vulnerable subjects. Evaluate the ethical aspects of one or both of these studies, paying special attention to the manner in which the subjects' heightened vulnerability was handled.

   a. Algase, D. L. et al. (1997). Estimates of stability of daily wandering behavior among cognitively impaired long-term care residents. *Nursing Research, 46,* 172–178.
   b. Flynn, L. (1997). The health practices of homeless women. *Nursing Research, 46,* 72–77.

4. In Chapter 4 in the textbook, two unethical studies were described (the study of syphilis among black men and the study in which live cancer cells were injected in elderly patients). Identify which ethical principles were transgressed in these studies.

_____

_____

_____

_____

5. A stipend of $15 was paid to the women who completed a questionnaire concerning their sexual histories and other topics in the following study:

Kenney, J. W., Reinholtz, C., & Angelini, P. J. (1998). Sexual abuse, sex before age 16, and high-risk behaviors of your females with sexually transmitted disease. *Journal of Obstetric, Gynecologic, and Neonatal Nursing, 27, 54–63.*

Read the introductory sections of the report and comment on the appropriateness of the stipend.

6. Comment on the risk/benefit ratio and other aspects of the following study, in which a mild form of deception was used:

Forrester, D. A. (1990). AIDS-related risk factors, medical diagnosis, do-not-resusictate orders and aggressiveness of nursing care. *Nursing Research, 39, 350-354.*

■ D. Application Exercises

1. Below is a brief description of the ethical aspects of a fictitious study, followed by a critique. Do you agree with the critique? Can you add other comments relevant to the ethical dimensions of the study (Box 4-2 of the textbook offers some guiding questions).

Fictitious Study. Starr (2000) conducted an in-depth study of nursing home patients to determine if their perceptions about personal control over decision making differed from the perceptions of the nursing staff. The investigator studied 25 nurse–patient dyads to determine whether there were differing perceptions and experiences regarding control over activities of daily living, such as arising, eating, and dressing. All of the nurses in the study were employed by the nursing home in which the patients resided. Because the nursing home had no IRB, Starr sought permission to conduct the study from the nursing home administrator. She also obtained the consent of the legal guardian or responsible family member of each patient. All study participants were fully informed about the nature of the study. The researcher assured the nurses and the legal guardians and family members of the patients of the confidentiality of the information and obtained their consent in writing. Data were gathered primarily through in-depth interviews with the patients and the nurses, at separate times. The researcher also observed interactions between the patients and nurses. The findings from the study showed that patients perceived that they had more control over all aspects of the activities of daily living (except eating) than the nurses perceived that they had. Excerpts from the interviews were used verbatim in the research report, but Starr did not divulge the location of the nursing home, and she used fictitious names for all participants.

Critique. Starr did a reasonably good job of adhering to basic ethical principles in the conduct of her research. She obtained written permission to conduct the study from the nursing home administrator, and she obtained informed consent from the nurse participants and the legal guardians or family members of the patients. The study participants were not put at risk in any way, and the patients who participated may actually have enjoyed the opportunity to have a conversation with the researcher. Starr also took appropriate steps to maintain the confidentiality of participants. It is still unclear, however, whether the patients knowingly and willingly participated in the research. Nursing home residents are a vulnerable group. They may not have been aware of their right to refuse to be interviewed without fear of repercussion. Starr could have enhanced the ethical aspects of the study by taking more vigorous steps to obtain the informed, voluntary consent of the nursing home residents or to exclude patients who could not reasonably be expected to understand the researcher's request. Given the vulnerability of the group, Starr might also have established her own review panel composed of peers and interested lay people to review the ethical dimensions of her project. Debriefing sessions with study participants would also have been appropriate.

2. Here is a brief description of ethical aspects of a fictitious study. Read the description and then respond to the questions that follow.

Fenton and Hammond (2001) investigated the behaviors of nursing students in crisis or emergency situations. The investigators were interested in comparing the behaviors of students from baccalaureate versus diploma programs to determine the adequacy of the preparation given to students in handling emergencies. Fifty students from both types of programs volunteered to participate in the study. The investigators wanted to observe reactions to crises as they might occur naturally, so the participants were not told the exact nature of the study. Each student was instructed to take the vital signs of a "patient," purportedly to evaluate the students' skills. The "patient," who was described as another student but who in fact was a confederate of the investigators, simulated an epileptic seizure while the vital signs were being taken. A research assistant, who was unaware of the purpose of the study and who did not know the educational background of the subjects, observed the timeliness and appropriateness of the students' responses to the situation through a one-way mirror. Participants were not required to fill out any forms that recorded their identities. Immediately after participation, the students were debriefed as to the true nature of the study and were paid a $10 stipend.

Consider the aspects of this study in terms of the issues discussed in this chapter. To assist you in your review, here are some guiding questions:

a. Were the study participants in this study at risk of physical or psychological harm? Were they at risk of exploitation?
b. Did the participants derive any benefits from their taking part in the study? Did the nursing community or society at large benefit? How would you assess the risk/benefit ratio?
c. Were the participants' rights to self-determination violated? Was there any coercion involved? Was full disclosure made before participation? Was informed consent given to participants and documented?
d. Were participants treated fairly? Was their right to privacy protected?
e. What ethical dilemmas does this study present? How, if at all, can the dilemmas be resolved? To what extent *were* they resolved?
f. What type of human subjects review would be appropriate for a study such as the one described?

3. Read one or more of the articles listed below. Respond to questions **a** through **f** from Question D.2 in terms of these actual research studies.

- Nesbitt, B. J., & Heidrich, S. M. (2000). Sense of coherence and illness appraisal in older women's quality of life. *Research in Nursing & Health, 23,* 25–34.

- Sayre, J. (2000). The patient's diagnosis: Explanatory models of mental illness. *Qualitative Health Research, 10,* 71–83.

- Sittner, B., Hudson, D., Grossman, C., & Gaston-Johansson, F. (1998). Adolescents' perceptions of pain during labor. *Clinical Nursing Research, 7,* 82–93.

- Wadas, T., & Hill, J. (1998). Is lidocaine infiltration during femoral sheath removal really necessary? *Heart & Lung, 27,* 31–36.

▪ E. Special Projects

1. Prepare a brief summary of a hypothetical study in which there are at least three major benefits to people participating in the study.

2. When the costs and benefits of a proposed study are essentially balanced, how should the researcher decide whether to proceed?

3. Skim the following research report, and draft an informed consent form for this study:

> Eden, B. M., Foreman, M. D., & Sisk, R. (1998). Delirium: Comparison of four predictive models is hospitalized critically ill elderly patients. *Applied Nursing Research, 11,* 27–35.

PART II

Preliminary Steps in the Research Process

CHAPTER 5

Scrutinizing Research Problems, Research Questions, and Hypotheses

■ A. Matching Exercises

1. Match each of the research problems in Set B with one of the statements in Set A. Indicate the letter corresponding to the appropriate response next to each statement in Set B.

SET A

a. Statement of purpose—qualitative study

b. Statement of purpose—quantitative study

c. Not a statement of purpose for a research study

SET B   **RESPONSES**

1. The purpose of this study is to test whether the removal of physical restraints affects behavioral changes in elderly patients.   _____

2. The purpose of this project is to facilitate the transition from hospital to home among women who have just given birth.   _____

3. The goal of this project is to explore the process by which an elderly person adjusts to placement in a nursing home.   _____

4. The investigation was designed to document the incidence and prevalence of smoking, alcohol use, and drug use among adolescents aged 12 to 14.   _____

5. The study's purpose was to describe the nature of touch used by parents in touching their preterm infants.   _____

6. The goal is to develop guidelines for spiritually related nursing interventions.   _____

SET B   **RESPONSES**

7. The purpose of this project is to examine the relationship between race/ethnicity and the use of over-the-counter medications.   _____

8. The purpose is to develop an in-depth understanding of patients' feelings of powerlessness in hospital settings.   _____

2. Match each of the statements in Set B with one of the terms in Set A. Indicate the letter corresponding to the appropriate response next to each statement in Set B.

SET A

a. Research hypothesis—directional
b. Research hypothesis—nondirectional
c. Null hypothesis
d. Not an hypothesis as stated

SET B   **RESPONSES**

1. First-born infants have higher concentrations of estrogens and progesterone in umbilical cord blood than do later-born infants.   _____

2. There is no relationship between participation in prenatal classes and the health outcomes of infants.   _____

3. Nursing students are increasingly interested in obtaining advanced degrees.   _____

4. Nurse practitioners have more job mobility than do other registered nurses.   _____

5. A person's age is related to his or her difficulty in accessing health care.   _____

6. Glaucoma can be effectively screened by means of tonometry.   _____

7. Increased noise levels result in increased anxiety among hospitalized patients.   _____

8. Media exposure regarding the health hazards of smoking is unrelated to the public's smoking habits.   _____

9. Patients' compliance with their medication regimens is related to their perceptions of the consequences of noncompliance.   _____

10. The primary reason that nurses participate in continuing education programs is for professional advancement.   _____

11. Baccalaureate, diploma, and associate degree nursing graduates differ with respect to technical and clinical skills acquired.   _____

12. A cancer patient's degree of hopefulness regarding the future is unrelated to his or her religiosity.   _____

13. The degree of attachment between infants and their mothers is associated with the infant's status as low birthweight or normal birthweight.   _____

14. The presence of homonymous hemianopia in stroke patients negatively affects their length of stay in hospital.   _____

15. Adjustment to hemodialysis does not vary by the patient's gender.   _____

▪ B. Completion Exercises

Write the words or phrases that correctly complete the sentences below.

1. A(n) _____ is a situation involving an enigmatic, puzzling, or disturbing condition that is of interest to a researcher.

2. A(n) _____ is a statement of the specific query the researcher seeks to answer.

3. The accomplishments a researcher hopes to achieve by conducting a study are referred to as the _____ or _____.

4. The five most common sources of ideas for research problems are _____, _____, _____, _____, and _____.

5. Research questions involving the essence, experience, process, or nature of some phenomenon would likely be addressed in a _____ _____ study.

6. Although it is desirable to have a statement of purpose placed early in a research report, the most typical location is at the end of the _____ _____.

7. Research hypotheses state a predicted _____
between variables.

8. A hypothesis involves a prediction regarding at least _____
_____ variables.

9. Hypotheses predict the effect of the _____
variable on the _____ variable.

10. A hypothesis that states a prediction regarding two or more independent
and two or more dependent variables is called a _____
or _____ hypothesis.

11. The _____ hypothesis states that there is no expected relationship among the research variables.

■ C. Study Questions

1. Define the following terms. Compare your definitions with those in Chapter 5 of the textbook or in the glossary.

a. Problem statement _____

_____.

b. Statement of purpose _____

_____.

c. Research question _____

_____.

d. Hypothesis _____

_____.

e. Simple hypothesis _____

_____.

f. Complex hypothesis _____

_____.

g. Nondirectional hypothesis _____

_____.

h. Null Hypothesis _____

_____.

i. Directional hypothesis _____

_____.

2. Below is a list of general topics that could be investigated. Develop at least one research question for each, making sure that some are questions that could be addressed through qualitative research and others are ones that could be addressed through quantitative research. (HINT: For quantitative research questions, think of these concepts as potential independent or dependent variables, then ask, "What might cause or affect this variable?" and "What might be the consequences or effects of this variable?" This should lead to some ideas for research questions.)

a. Patient comfort _____

_____.

b. Psychiatric patients' readmission rates _____

_____.

c. Anxiety in hospitalized children _____

_____.

d. Elevated blood pressure _____

_____.

e. Incidence of sexually transmitted diseases (STDs) _____

_____.

f. Patient cooperativeness in the recovery room _____

_____.

g. Caregiver stress _____

_____.

h. Mother–infant bonding _____

_____.

i. Menstrual irregularities _____

_____.

3. Below is a list of research questions and statements of purpose. Transform those stated in the interrogative form (as research questions) to the declarative form (as statements of purpose), and vice versa.

Original Version   *Transformed Version*

a. Can a program of nursing counseling   _____
    affect sexual readjustment among   _____
    women after a hysterectomy?   _____

b. The purpose of the research is to   _____
    study the lived experience of parents   _____
    whose young children have died   _____
    of cancer.   _____

c. What are the sequelae of an   _____
    inadequately maintained sterile   _____
    environment for tracheal suctioning?   _____

d. What are the cues nurses use to   _____
    determine pain in infants?   _____

e. The purpose of the study is to   _____
    investigate the effect of an AIDS   _____
    education workshop on teenagers'   _____
    understanding of AIDS and the   _____
    HIV virus.   _____

f. The purpose of the research is to fully _____
    describe patients' responses to   _____
    transfer from a coronary care unit.   _____

g. What effect does the presence of the   _____
    father in the delivery room have on   _____
    the mother's satisfaction with the   _____
    childbirth experience?   _____

h. The purpose of the study is to explore _____
    why some women fail to perform   _____
    breast self-examination regularly.   _____

i. What is the long-term child-develop-   _____
    ment effect of maternal heroin   _____
    addiction during pregnancy?   _____

j. The purpose of the research is to study _____

    the effect of spermicides on the _____

    physiologic development of the fetus. _____

4. Below are five nondirectional hypotheses. Restate each one as a directional hypothesis.

Nondirectional	*Directional*

  a. Tactile stimulation is associated _____

    with comparable physiological _____

    arousal as verbal stimulation among _____

    infants with congenital heart disease. _____

  b. Nurses and patients differ in terms _____

    of the relative importance they attach _____

    to having the patients' physical _____

    versus emotional needs met. _____

  c. Type of nursing care (primary versus _____

    team) is unrelated to patient _____

    satisfaction with the care received. _____

  d. The incidence of decubitus ulcers is _____

    related to the frequency of turning _____

    patients. _____

  e. Nurses administer the same amount _____

    of narcotic analgesics to male and _____

    female patients. _____

5. Below are five simple hypotheses. Change each one to a complex hypothesis by adding either a dependent or independent variable.

Simple Hypothesis	*Complex Hypothesis*

  a. First-time blood donors experience _____

    greater stress during the donation _____

    than donors who have given blood _____

    previously. _____

b. Nurses who initiate more conversation with patients are rated as more effective in their nursing care by patients than those who initiate less conversation.

_____
_____
_____
_____
_____

c. Surgical patients who give high ratings to the informativeness of nursing communications experience less preoperative stress than do patients who give low ratings.

_____
_____
_____
_____
_____

d. Appendectomy patients whose peritoneums are drained with a Penrose drain will experience more peritoneal infection than patients who are not drained.

_____
_____
_____
_____
_____

e. Women who give birth by cesarean section are more likely to experience postpartum depression than women who give birth vaginally.

_____
_____
_____
_____

6. In study questions 4 and 5 above, 10 research hypotheses were provided. Identify the independent and dependent variables in each.

INDEPENDENT VARIABLE(S)   **DEPENDENT VARIABLE(S)**

4a _____   _____

4b _____   _____

4c _____   _____

4d _____   _____

4e _____   _____

5a _____   _____

5b _____   _____

5c _____   _____

5d_____   _____

5e _____   _____

7. Below are five statements that are *not* research hypotheses as currently stated. Suggest modifications to these statements that would make them testable research hypotheses.

Original Statement	*Hypothesis*
a. Relaxation therapy is effective in reducing hypertension.	
b. The use of bilingual health care staff produces high utilization rates of health care facilities by ethnic minorities.	
c. Nursing students are affected in their choice of clinical specialization by interactions with nursing faculty.	
d. Sexually active teenagers have a high rate of using male methods of contraception.	
e. In-use intravenous solutions become contaminated within 48 hours.	

■ D. Application Exercises

1. Below is a brief description of a research problem for a fictitious study, followed by a critique. Do you agree with the critique? Can you add other comments relevant to issues discussed in Chapter 5 of the textbook? (Box 5-1 offers some guiding questions.)

   Fictitious Study. Clemente (2000) was interested in studying non-verbal communication between nurses and patients. After some preliminary reading and discussions with colleagues, she decided to focus on touch as the medium of communication. She described her research question as follows: Does the amount of touching nurses give to patients affect the patients' recovery? Based on Clemente's readings regarding the effects of touch, she formulated the following hypotheses:

- Without specific instruction regarding touching as a therapeutic form of communication, nurses do not engage in much touching behavior.
- The more nurses touch their patients, the higher the patients' morale.
- The greater the amount of physical contact between nurses and patients, the greater is the likelihood that the patients will comply with nurses' instructions, and the fewer the number of days of hospitalization.

Critique. This example illustrates how the researcher narrowed and refined a broad topic of interest—nonverbal communication— and developed several research hypotheses in a series of steps. Those steps involved reviewing the literature, consulting with other nurses, identifying a specific area of interest for investigation, developing a research question, and finally, formulating the research hypotheses.

Using the criteria presented in this chapter, we can evaluate Clemente's research question and hypotheses. The research question appears to meet the criterion of significance: There are some tangible and important applications that can be made of the findings for the nursing profession. The question does not deal with a moral or ethical issue and meets the criterion for researchability. Without further information, we cannot judge the feasibility of the study, but presumably the study could be accomplished without undue constraints.

One difficulty, however, is that the leap between the research question and the hypotheses is a great one. The first hypothesis, though thematically related to the research question, does not address the issue of patient recovery at all. The second hypothesis is also tenuously connected to the problem statement; improved patient morale is undoubtedly a desirable outcome, but it is not really an acceptable way to operationalize speed of recovery. The final hypothesis (a complex hypothesis) is an appropriate translation of the formal problem statement into hypothesis form. Here, the researcher is defining patient recovery in terms of compliance with instructions and days spent in the hospital.

Aside from the gap between the research question and the hypotheses, there are additional problems with the hypotheses. The first hypothesis is untestable because it fails to state a predicted relationship between two variables. What criterion can we use to decide what "much touching" is? This hypothesis could be tested if rephrased in the following way: Nurses who receive instruction on the therapeutic value of touching will engage in more touching of patients than those who do not receive instruction.

In summary, there are many laudable features of Clemente's efforts. She has identified a significant, researchable topic and formulated some testable hypotheses; however, several modifications to the research question and hypotheses are in order.

2. Here is a brief description of certain aspects of a fictitious study. Read the description and then respond to the questions that follow.

Montanari (2001) was interested in studying the notes made by various members of the health care team on patients' hospital charts. The investigator was concerned with several aspects of the chart in terms of its communication potential to various hospital personnel. She began her project with some general questions, such as: Are the nurses' entries on the patient chart used by other staff? Who is most likely to read nurses' entries on the patient chart? Are there particular types of medical conditions that encourage staff utilization of nurses' entries? Do particular types of entries encourage utilization?

Montanari proceeded to reflect on her own experiences and observations relative to these issues and reviewed the literature to find whether other researchers had these problems. Based on her review and reflections, Montanari developed the following hypotheses:

- Nursing notes on patients' charts are referred to infrequently by hospital personnel.
- Physicians refer to nursing notes on the patients' charts less frequently than do other personnel.
- The use of nursing notes by physicians is related to the location of the notes on the chart.
- Nurses perceive that nursing notes are referred to less frequently than they are in fact referred to.
- Nursing notes are more likely to be referred to by hospital personnel if the patient has been hospitalized for more than 5 days than if the patient has been hospitalized for 5 days or fewer.

Review and critique the hypotheses and the process of developing them. Suggest alternative wordings or supplementary hypotheses. To assist you, here are some guiding questions:

a. Are all the hypotheses testable as stated? What changes (if any) are needed to make all the hypotheses testable?

b. Are the hypotheses all consistent in format and style? That is, are they directional, nondirectional, or stated in the null form? Suggest changes, if appropriate, that would make them consistent.

c. Are the hypotheses reasonable (i.e., logical and consistent with your own experience and observations)? Are the hypotheses significant (i.e., do they have the potential to contribute to the nursing profession)?

d. Based on the general problem that the researcher identified, can you generate additional hypotheses that could be tested? Can you suggest modifications to the hypotheses to make them complex rather than simple (i.e., introduce additional independent or dependent variables)?

3. Below are several suggested research articles. Read the introductory sections of one or more of these articles and identify the research questions and hypotheses. Respond to parts **a** to **d** of Question D.2 in terms of these actual research studies.

- Bull, M. J., Hansen, H. E., & Gross, C. R. (2000). A professional-patient partnership model of discharge planning with elders hospitalized with heart failure. *Applied Nursing Research, 13,* 19–28.

- Lutenbacher, M., & Hall, L.A. (1998). The effects of psychosocial factors on parenting attitudes of low-income, single mothers with young children. *Nursing Research, 47,* 25–34.

- Preston, D. B., Forti, E. M., Kassab, C., & Koch, P. B. (2000). Personal and social determinants of rural nurses' willingness to care for persons with AIDS. *Research in Nursing & Health, 23,* 67–78.

- Ronen, T., & Abraham, Y. (1996). Retention control training in the treatment of younger versus older enuretic children. *Nursing Research, 45,* 78–86.

- Trinkoff, A. M., Zhou, Q., Storr, C. L., & Soeken, K. L. (2000). Workplace access, negative proscriptions, job strain, and substance use in registered nurses. *Nursing Research, 49,* 83–90.

4. Another brief summary of a fictitious study follows. Read the summary and then respond to the questions that follow.

Zilbermann (2001), herself an asthmatic, noticed that when she experienced dyspnea she had a tendency to stop moving. A preliminary search of the literature on dyspnea suggested that there was relatively little research on how people with a chronic pulmonary disease react to and cope with the sensation of dyspnea. She conducted a qualitative study guided by a very general question—how is dyspnea experienced by people with a chronic pulmonary disorder? As she began to discuss this issue with study participants, Zilbermann noticed that people with the three most common types of pulmonary disease—asthma, emphysema, and bronchitis—had developed somewhat different strategies for coping with dyspnea. On the basis of her in-depth interviews (and her observations of several study participants experiencing dyspnea), her final research questions evolved into the following:

- What are the coping strategies used by patients with different chronic pulmonary diseases to deal with dyspnea?
- What aspects of the dyspnea experience trigger different coping mechanisms?
- What are the *patterns* of coping mechanism used by patients (i.e., what strategies are used in what order)?

Review and critique the researcher's research questions. To assist you, here are some guiding questions.
a. Are the research questions clearly articulated?
b. Comment on the significance of the research questions for the nursing profession.
c. Does the research question appear to be well-suited to a qualitative approach?
d. Does the researcher's development of her research questions appear to have followed an appropriate process?
e. Are the research questions worded properly?

5. Below are several suggested research articles. Read the introductory sections of one or more of these articles and identify the research questions. Respond to parts **a** to **e** of Question D.4 in terms of these actual research studies.

- Davis, R. E. (2000). Refugee experiences and Southeast Asian women's mental health. *Western Journal of Nursing Research, 22,* 144–168.
- Hupcey, J. E. (1998). Establishing the nurse-family relationship in the intensive care unit. *Western Journal of Nursing Research, 20,* 180–194.
- King, G., Stewart, D., King, S., & Law, M. (2000). Organizational characteristics and issues affecting the longevity of self-help groups for parents of children with special needs. *Qualitative Health Research, 10,* 225–241.
- Paterson, B., & Thorne, S. (2000). Expert decision making in relation to unanticipated blood glucose levels. *Research in Nursing & Health, 23,* 147–157.

■ E. Special Projects

1. Think of your clinical experience as a student or practicing nurse. Consider some aspect of your work that you particularly enjoy. Is there anything about that part of your work that puzzles, intrigues, or frustrates you? Can you conceive of any procedure, practice, or information that would improve the quality of your work in that area or improve the care you provide? Ask yourself a series of similar questions until a general problem area emerges. Narrow the problem area until you have a workable research problem statement. Assess the problem in terms of the criteria of significance, researchability, feasibility, and interest to you.

2. Below are two sets of variables. Select a variable from each set to generate directional hypotheses. In other words, use one variable in Set A as the independent variable and one variable in Set B as the dependent variable (or vice versa), and make a prediction about the relationship between the two.* Generate five hypotheses in this fashion. Then assess the hypotheses generated in terms of significance, testability, and interest to you.

SET A	**SET B**
Body temperature	Patient satisfaction with nursing care
Patients' level of hopefulness	Regular versus no exercise
Attitudes toward death	Infant Apgar score
Frequency of medications	Patients' gender
Delivery by nurse midwife versus physician	Effectiveness of nursing care
Participation in continuing education courses	Patients' capacity for self-care
Years of nursing experience	Patients' compliance with nursing instructions
Amount of interaction between nurses and patients' families	Amount of analgesics administered
Preoperative anxiety levels	Breastfeeding duration
Patients' amount of privacy during hospitalization	Nurses' empathy Patients' pulse rates
Smoking status (smokes versus does not smoke)	Patients' length of stay in hospital
Recidivism in a psychiatric hospital	

---

*As one example: Pregnant women who smoke will give birth to babies with lower Apgar scores than women who do not smoke.

CHAPTER 6

Reviewing the Research Literature

■ A. Matching Exercise

1. Match each of the statements in Set B with one or more of the terms in Set A. Indicate the letter corresponding to the appropriate response next to each entry in Set B.

SET A

a. Electronic databases
b. Print indexes
c. Abstract journals
d. None of the above

SET B   RESPONSES

1. Can be accessed only by librarians or information specialists.   _____

2. CINAHL.   _____

3. Can be searched by subjects/keywords.   _____

4. Is an especially efficient means of accessing references.   _____

5. Does not include a summary of research studies.   _____

6. Are universally available in hospitals and nursing schools.   _____

7. Has mapping capabilities.   _____

8. MEDLINE.   _____

9. Each volume covers a specified time period.   _____

10. Manual searches use these.   _____

■ B. Completion Exercises

Write the words or phrases that correctly complete the sentences below.

1. For nurses, the most widely used electronic database is _____
_____.

2. Most electronic searches are likely to begin with a _____
_____ search.

3. An electronic search that looks for a topic or keyword as it appears in
the text fields of a record is referred to as a _____
search.

4. The two major types of print resources for a bibliographic search are
_____ and_____.

5. In the context of the research literature, a _____
source is a description of a study written by the researchers who conducted it.

6. The most important type of information to be included in a written research review is _____.

7. Quantity of references is less important in a good literature review than
the _____ of the references.

8. The written literature review should paraphrase materials and use a minimum of _____.

9. The literature review should make clear not only what is known about a
problem but also any _____ in the research.

10. The review should conclude with a _____.

11. The review should be written in a language of _____,
in keeping with the limitations of available methods.

■ C. Study Questions

1. Define the following terms. Compare your definition with the definition
in Chapter 6 of the textbook or in the glossary.

   a. Literature review _____

   _____.

   b. On-line search _____

   _____.

c. Mapping _____

_____.

d. Key word _____

_____.

e. Abstract journal _____

_____.

f. Primary source _____

_____.

g. Secondary source _____

_____.

2. Below are fictitious excerpts from research literature reviews. Each excerpt has a stylistic problem. Change each sentence to make it acceptable stylistically.

Original   *Revised*

a. Most elderly people do not   _____
   eat a balanced diet.   _____

b. Patient characteristics have a   _____
   significant impact on nursing   _____
   workload.   _____

c. A child's conception of appropriate _____
   sick role behavior changes as the   _____
   child grows older.   _____

d. Home birth poses many potential   _____
   dangers.   _____

e. Multiple sclerosis results in   _____
   considerable anxiety to the family _____
   of the patients.   _____

f. Studies have proved that most   _____
   nurses prefer not to work the night _____
   shift.   _____

Original   *Revised*

  g. Life changes are the major cause

     of stress in adults.

  h. Stroke rehabilitation programs are

     most effective when they involve

     the patients' families.

  i. It has been proved that psychiatric

     outpatients have higher than

     average rates of accidental deaths

     and suicides.

  j. Nursing faculty are increasingly

     involved in conducting their own

     research.

  k. The traditional pelvic examination

     is sufficiently unpleasant to many

     women that they avoid having the

     examination.

  l. It is known that most tonsillectomies

     performed three decades ago were

     unnecessary.

  m. Few smokers seriously try to break

     the smoking habit.

  n. Severe cutaneous burns often result

     in hemorrhagic gastric erosions.

3. Below are several problem statements. Indicate one or more keywords
that you would use to begin a literature search on this topic.

Problem Statement	*Key Words*
a. How effective are nurse practitioners compared with pediatricians with respect to telephone management of acute pediatric illness?	_____ _____ _____ _____ _____
b. Does contingency contracting improve patient compliance with a treatment regimen?	_____ _____ _____
c. What is the decision-making process for a woman considering having an abortion?	_____ _____ _____
d. Is the amount of money a person spends on food related to the adequacy of nutrient intake?	_____ _____ _____
e. Is rehabilitation after spinal cord injury affected by the age and occupation of the patient?	_____ _____ _____
f. Does the leadership style of head nurses affect the job tension and job performance of the nursing staff?	_____ _____ _____
g. What is the course of appetite loss among cancer patients undergoing chemotherapy?	_____ _____ _____
h. What is the effect of alcohol skin preparation before insulin injection on the incidence of local and systemic infection?	_____ _____ _____

Problem Statement	Key Words
i. Are bottle-fed babies introduced to solid foods sooner than breastfed babies?	_____ _____ _____
j. Do children raised on vegetarian diets have different growth patterns than other children?	_____ _____ _____

4. Read the Keuter et al. (2000) study entitled "Nurses' job satisfaction and organizational climate in a dynamic work environment," which appeared in *Applied Nursing Research, 13*, 46–49. Write a summary of the research problem, methods, findings, and conclusions of the study. Your summary should be capable of serving as notes for a review of the literature on nurses' job satisfaction in relation to organizational climate.

■ D. Application Exercises

1. Below is a brief description of the literature review from a fictitious study by Edelman (2000), followed by a critique. Do you agree with the critique? Can you add other comments relevant to issues relating to a literature review, as discussed in Chapter 6 of the textbook? (Box 6-1 offers some guiding questions.)

   Fictitious Literature Review. There is now abundant evidence in the medical and epidemiologic literature that adolescents are at especially high risk of pregnancy complications, giving birth to low-birth-weight infants, and neonatal deaths (Hillard, 1992; Travis, 1986; Brown, 1989).* Relatively few studies, however, have examined the health status of children born to adolescent mothers after the first few weeks of life. The limited data that are available suggest that children of young mothers continue to be at a disadvantage throughout their infancy and later childhood. For example, Bradley and Lewis (1991) reported that the health of infants born to African American teenaged mothers was worse than that for infants of older African American mothers; particular problems were noted with respect to hypoglycemia, respiratory distress syndrome, pneumonia, and seizures. Hughes (1991), in her intensive study of young-parent

---

*The citations are fictitious.

families, reported an extremely high incidence of health problems among the infants: One-fifth had been hospitalized by the time they were 18 months old. According to Tilmon (1989), "These young women are simply not capable of attending to the needs of their children until these problems are so severe they require hospitalization" (p. 315).

Other investigators have proved that accidents and injuries are more prevalent among infants born to teenaged mothers. For example, Wright (1990) reported that the risk of infant accidental death was highest among mothers between 15 and 19 years of age. Similarly, Kestecher and Dickinson (1993) found that the most important difference in the health status between 3-year-old children with teenaged mothers and those with older mothers was the high incidence of injuries and burns to children of younger mothers.

Few empirical studies have attempted to unravel the factors that might lead to impaired health among the children born to younger mothers. The purpose of this study was to further our understanding of the factors that might lead to greater health problems and less appropriate use of health care among children born to adolescent mothers.

Critique. For the most part, Edelman appears to have done a fairly good job of organizing and briefly summarizing information about the effect of maternal age on an infant's health status. The research cited appears to be relevant to the research problem, and Edelman seems to have relied on primary sources. Without doing a literature review ourselves, it would be difficult to know whether this review is accurate and thorough. We do know, however, that most of the references were fairly old. None of the research cited was conducted in the three years preceding publication of Edelman's report. It is therefore likely that this review excluded other more recent research on this topic—research that might have made a difference in Edelman's conclusions and formulation of the problem.

Edelman's review can also be criticized for being fairly superficial. True, in journal articles, it is common for researchers to be succinct and to cite only the most important relevant studies. It would have been helpful, however, for Edelman to make a statement about the believability of the previous research findings based on an assessment of the quality and integrity of the studies.

Two other points about the literature review merit comment. The first is that Edelman inappropriately claimed that prior studies "proved" that accidents and injuries are more prevalent among infants of young mothers. The word "proved" should be changed to found or some other tentative phrasing. Second, there is an irrelevant and subjective quotation buried in a review that otherwise seems to be objective and neutral. The quote by Tilmon does not belong in this review. Edelman could have introduced the quote this way: "Findings such as these have led some authorities to speculate about whether young mothers are developmentally prepared to handle the parenting role. For example, Tilmon (1979), who chaired a panel on high-risk infants, made the comment . . ."

2. Below is an excerpt from a fictitious literature review by Bokan (2001) dealing with pelvic inflammatory disease. Read the literature review and then respond to the questions that follow.

There are no universally accepted criteria for defining pelvic inflammatory disease (PID) or for categorizing its severity. Furthermore, PID does not exhibit uniformity in its clinical features. Etiologically, cases of acute PID can be divided on the basis of those caused by *Neisseria gonorrhoeae,* those caused by nongonococcal bacteria, and those caused by a combination of both. Eschenbach and his colleagues (1990) reported that about half of the women with PID whom they examined had gonococcal infections. Eschenbach (1989) noted that "this difference in etiological agents may explain the clinical differences between the gonococcal and nongonococcal PID. The latter may appear less acute and may not demonstrate many of the well-defined clinical features associated with gonorrhea" (p. 148). Both gonococcal and nongonococcal PID may result in subsequent obstruction of the fallopian tubes, which is among the most common causes of infertility in women. Because fertilized eggs remain in the fallopian tubes for about three days, they must provide nourishment for the developing zygote. Thus, even a tube that is not completely blocked, but which is severely damaged, can contribute to infertility.

Westrom (1995), in a study of women treated for PID, proved that PID has an impact on subsequent fertility. A sample of 415 women with laparoscopically confirmed PID were reviewed after 9.5 years and compared with 100 control subjects who had never been treated for PID. Among the 415 women who had had PID, 88 (21.2%) were involuntarily childless; of these 88, the failure to conceive was due to tubal obstruction in 72 cases (82%). A total of 263 of the 415 subjects (63.4%) had become pregnant. In the control group, only three women (3%) were involuntarily childless.

Westrom's study also revealed a relationship between infertility and the number of PID infections. Tubal occlusion was diagnosed after one infection in 32 women (12.8%); after two infections in 22 cases (35.5%); and after three or more infections in 18 cases (75.0%). Of the 415 women with acute PID in Westrom's sample, 94 (22.7%) experienced more than one infection. Evidence from other studies confirms that a large percentage of women with PID have a history of previous PID and that recurrent PID usually has a nongonococcal etiology (Jacobson & Westrom, 1988; Ringrose, 1994; Eschenbach, 1989).

The number of women affected by PID annually in the United States is unknown and difficult to estimate. According to Rose (1996), Eschenbach and colleagues used data from the National Disease and Therapeutic Index Study and the Hospital Record Study to estimate that over 500,000 cases of PID occurred annually in the United States in the early 1980s. The information from the Hospital Record Study indicated that a mean of over 160,000 patients with PID were hospitalized annually from 1980 through 1983.

Critique this literature review regarding the points made in Chapter 6 of the textbook. To assist you in this task, here are some guiding questions:

a. Is the review well organized? Does the author skip from theme to theme in a disjointed way, or is there a logic to the order of presentation of materials?

b. Is the content of the review appropriate? Did the author use secondary sources when a primary source was available? Are all the references relevant, or does the inclusion of some material appear contrived? Do you have a sense that the author was thorough in uncovering all the relevant materials? Do the references seem outdated? Is there an overdependence on opinion articles and/or anecdotes? Are prior studies merely summarized, or are shortcomings discussed? Does the author indicate what is not known as well as what is?

c. Does the style seem appropriate for a research review? Does the review seem biased or laden with subjective opinions? Is there too little paraphrasing and too much quoting? Does the author use appropriately tentative language in describing the results of earlier studies?

3. Read the literature review section in one of the articles listed below. Critique the review, applying questions a through c from Question D.2 above.

- Brown, J. K., Whittemore, K. T., & Knapp, T. R. (2000). Is arm span an accurate measure of height in young and middle-age adults? *Clinical Nursing Research, 9,* 84–94.

- Fontana, J. A. (2000). The energy costs of a modified form of T'ai Chi exercise. *Nursing Research, 49,* 91–96.

- Meininger, J. C., Hayman, L. L., Coates, P. M., & Gallagher, P. R. (1998). Genetic and environmental influences on cardiovascular disease risk factors in adolescents. *Nursing Research, 47,* 11–18.

- Thomas, K. A. (2000). Differential effects of breast- and formula-feeding on preterm infants' sleep-wake patterns. *Journal of Obstetric, Gynecologic, and Neonatal Nursing, 29,* 145–152.

- Thorne, S. E., & Radford, M. J. (1998). A comparative longitudinal study of gastrostomy devices in children. *Western Journal of Nursing Research, 20,* 145–165.

▪ E. Special Projects

1. Read the literature review section from a research article appearing in a nursing journal in the early 1990s (some possibilities are suggested below). Search the literature for more recent research on the topic of the article and update the original researchers' review section. Don't forget to incorporate in your review the findings from the cited research article itself! Here are some possible articles:

- Bonheur, B., & Young, S. W. (1991). Exercise as a health-promoting lifestyle choice. *Applied Nursing Research, 4,* 2–6.

- Long, K. A., & Boik, R. J. (1993). Predicting alcohol use in rural children. *Nursing Research, 42,* 79–86.

- Morse, J. M., & Hutchinson, E. (1991). Releasing restraints: Providing safe care for the elderly. *Research in Nursing & Health, 14,* 382–396.

- Quinn, M. M. (1991). Attachment between mothers and their down syndrome infants. *Western Journal of Nursing Research, 13,* 382–396.

- Shapiro, C. R. (1993). Nurses' judgments of pain in term and preterm newborns. *Journal of Obstetric, Gynecologic, and Neonatal Nursing, 22,* 41–48.

2. Select one of the problem statements from Question C.3. Conduct a literature search and identify five to ten relevant references. Compare your references with those of your classmates in terms of relevance, recency, and type of information provided.

CHAPTER 7

Examining Theoretical Frameworks

■ A. Matching Exercises

1. Match each statement from Set B with one of the phrases in Set A. Indicate the letter corresponding to your response next to each of the statements in Set B.

SET A

a. Classic theory
b. Conceptual framework/model
c. Schematic model
d. Neither a, b, nor c
e. a, b, and c

SET B   **RESPONSES**

1. Makes minimal use of language.   _____

2. Uses concepts as building blocks.   _____

3. Is essential in the conduct of good research.   _____

4. Can be used as a basis for generating hypotheses.   _____

5. Can be proved through empirical testing.   _____

6. Indicates a system of propositions that assert
   relationships among variables.   _____

7. Consists of interrelated concepts organized in a rational
   scheme but does not specify formal relationships
   among the concepts.   _____

8. Exists in nature and is awaiting scientific discovery. _____

2. Match each model from Set B with one of the theorists in Set A. Indicate the letter corresponding to your response next to each of the statements in Set B.

SET A

a. Orem

b. Pender

c. Roy

d. Becker

e. Lazarus-Folkman

f. Mishel

SET B   **RESPONSES**

1. Adaptation Model   _____

2. Health Belief Model   _____

3. Uncertainty in Illness Theory   _____

4. Model of Self-Care   _____

5. Theory of Stress and Coping   _____

6. Health Promotion Model   _____

■ B. Completion Exercises

Write the words or phrases that correctly complete the sentences below.

1. Theories are not found by scientists, they are _____
   _____.

2. Deductions from theories are referred to as _____
   _____.

3. A _____ is the conceptual
   underpinning of a study.

4. Most of the conceptualizations of nursing practice would be called
   _____.

5. Schematic models attempt to represent reality with a minimal use of
   _____.

6. The four central concepts of conceptual models in nursing are
   _____, _____,
   _____, and _____.

7. The basic intellectual process underlying theory development is
   _____.

8. The acronym HPM stands for the _____.

9. Theoretical frameworks from nonnursing disciplines are sometimes referred to as _____.

10. Many qualitative researchers seek to develop a _____ _____ theory, a conceptualization of a phenomenon rooted in the researcher's observations.

■ C. Study Questions

1. Define the following terms. Compare your definitions with those in the glossary or in Chapter 7 of the textbook.

   a. Descriptive theory _____

   _____

   b. Macrotheory _____

   _____

   c. Middle-range theory _____

   _____

   d. Conceptual framework _____

   _____

   e. Conceptual definition _____

   _____

   f. Schematic model _____

   _____

   g. Statistical model _____

   _____

2. Read some recent issues of a nursing research journal. Identify at least three different theories cited by nurse researchers in these research reports.

   _____

   _____

   _____

   _____

   _____

3. Choose one of the conceptual frameworks of nursing that were described in this chapter. Develop a research hypothesis based on this framework.

_____

_____

_____

_____

_____

4. Select one of the research questions/problems listed in Question C.3, Chapter 5 of this Study Guide. Could your selected problem be developed within one of the nursing frameworks discussed in this chapter? Defend your answer.

_____

_____

_____

_____

_____

▪ D. Application Exercises

1. Pfeil (2000) conducted a study to examine factors related to the health and health care of children born to adolescent mothers. Below is a brief description of the conceptual framework used in this fictitious study, followed by a critique. Do you agree with the critique? Can you add other comments relevant to issues relating to the conceptual framework, as discussed in Chapter 7 of the textbook? (Box 7-1 offers some guiding questions.)

Fictitious Conceptual Framework. There is now abundant evidence in the medical and epidemiologic literature that adolescents are at especially high risk of pregnancy complications and that their infants have a higher-than-average rate of low-birth-weight and neonatal death. Relatively few studies, however, have examined the health status of children born to adolescent mothers after the first few weeks of life. The limited data that are available suggest that children of young mothers continue to be at a disadvantage throughout their infancy and later childhood. The purpose of this study was to further our understanding of the factors that might lead to greater health problems and less appropriate use of health care among children born to adolescent mothers.

The theoretical framework for this study was the Health Belief Model (HBM). This model postulates that health-seeking behavior is influenced by the perceived threat posed by a health problem and the perceived value of actions designed to reduce the threat (Becker, 1978). Within the HBM, perceived susceptibility refers to a person's perception that a health problem is personally relevant. It is hypothesized that young mothers are developmentally unable to perceive their own (or their infant's) susceptibility to health risk accurately. Furthermore, adolescent mothers are hypothesized to be less likely, because of their developmental immaturity, to perceive accurately the severity of their infants' health problems and less likely to assess accurately the benefit of appropriate interventions than older mothers. Finally, teenaged mothers are expected to evaluate less accurately the costs (which, in the HBM, include the complexity, duration, accessibility, and financial costs) of securing treatment. In summary, the HBM provides an excellent vehicle for testing the mechanisms through which children of young mothers are at higher-than-average risk of severe health problems and are less likely to receive appropriate health care.

Critique. The theoretical basis for Pfeil's study was a nonnursing model that has frequently been applied to problems relating to health care use. This model appears to have provided an appropriate conceptual basis for the study. Although Pfeil might have provided somewhat more information regarding features of the HBM, she did explain the HBM sufficiently to clarify the basis for her hypotheses. Her hypotheses are clearly linked to the model and appear to be logically related to the problem at hand.

Previous research had yielded descriptive information suggesting that children born to teenaged mothers are at higher risk than other children for health problems and inadequate health care. By basing this research on the HBM, Pfeil was attempting to explain why this might be so. She hypothesized that the differences between the children of older and younger mothers reflect the younger mothers' appraisals of their children's needs and of the value of obtaining treatment. By operationalizing the key concepts in the HBM (e.g., perceived susceptibility, perceived severity of the illness, perceived cost of securing treatment), Pfeil's hypotheses can be put to an empirical test. If Pfeil found differences between older and young mothers in their appraisals of their children's health care needs, progress would have been made toward explaining differences in the children's health outcomes. If, however, Pfeil found no differences in mothers' appraisals, another researcher interested in the same problem would have to evaluate whether a different conceptual framework might be more productive in helping to explain differences in children's health and health care, or whether Pfeil failed—through her research design decisions—to test the HBM adequately.

2. Below is a description of the conceptual framework for a fictitious study. Read the summary and then respond to the questions that follow.

Joyce (1999) developed a study derived from Rotter's social learning theory. Social learning theory postulates that human behaviors are contingent on the individual's expectancy that a particular behavior will be reinforced (rewarded). A key concept is locus of control, which is conceptualized as the degree to which a person perceives that rewards are a function of his or her own actions as opposed to external forces. Internal controllers are those who perceive themselves and their behavior as the major determinants of the reinforcement, while external controllers are those who tend to see little, if any, relationship between their own actions and subsequent reinforcement.

Joyce hypothesized that people with an internal locus-of-control orientation would be more likely to engage in preventive health care activities than those with an external orientation. As a rationale for this hypothesis, she reasoned that "internal" people see themselves as capable of controlling health outcomes, while externally oriented people see forces outside of their control as the major determinants of health outcomes; the "externals" are, therefore, less likely to engage in preventive health care behaviors. To test her hypothesis, Joyce operationalized "willingness to engage in preventive health care activities" as enrollment in a health maintenance organization (HMO) among a group of employees who were offered a choice between a traditional medical benefits package and HMO membership. Five hundred employees hired by a large industrial firm were administered a test that measured locus of control as part of the application process. Each new employee was offered a choice between the two medical programs. The 187 employees who chose HMO membership were found to have significantly higher (i.e., more internal) scores on the locus-of-control measure than the 313 employees who elected the traditional medical plan, thereby supporting Joyce's hypothesis.

Review and critique the above study, particularly with respect to its theoretical basis. To assist you in your critique, here are some guiding questions:

a. Examine the study variables. To what extent are they congruent with the conceptual perspective of the study's theoretical framework? Can you offer any suggestions for a different theoretical basis than the one used?

b. Do the hypotheses and research methods flow naturally from the theoretical framework, or does the link between them seem contrived?

c. In what way, if any, did the use of a theory enhance the value of this study? Compare the meaningfulness of the study as described with what it would have been had the same hypothesis been tested in the absence of a theory.

d. In what way, if any, did the outcome of the study affect the value of the theory? If the outcome had been different (e.g., no differences, or differences opposite to those predicted), what effect would that have had on the theory?

3. Read the introductory sections of one of the actual research studies cited below. Apply questions a through d from Question D.2 to one of these studies.

- Nesbitt, B. J., & Heidrich, S. M. (2000). Sense of coherence and illness appraisal in older women's quality of life. *Research in Nursing & Health, 23,* 25-34.

- Popkess-Vawter, S., Wendel, S., Schmoll, S., & O'Connell, K. (1998). Overeating, reversal theory and weight cycling. *Western Journal of Nursing Research, 20,* 67–83.

- Sowell, R., Moneyham, L., Hennessy, M., Guillory, J., Demi, A., & Seals, B. (2000). Spiritual activities as a resistance resource for women with human immunodeficiency virus. *Nursing Research, 49,* 73–82.

- Stein, K. F., Roeser, R., & Markus, H. R. (1998). Self-schemas and possible selves as predictors and outcomes of risky behavior in adolescents. *Nursing Research, 47,* 96–105.

- Swanson, K. M. (1999). Effects of caring, measurement, and time on miscarriage impact and women's well-being. *Nursing Research, 48,* 288–297.

■ E. Special Projects

1. One proposition of reinforcement theory is that *if* a behavior is rewarded (reinforced), *then* the behavior will be repeated (learned). Based on this theory and on your observation of behaviors in health settings or schools of nursing, suggest three nursing research problem statements.

2. Develop a researchable problem statement based on Orem's Model of Self Care or Pender's Health Promotion Model (Figure 7-1).

PART III

Designs for Nursing Research

CHAPTER 8

Understanding Quantitative Research Design

■ A. Matching Exercises

1. Match each problem statement from Set B with one (or more) of the phrases from Set A that indicates a potential reason for using a nonexperimental approach. Indicate the letter(s) corresponding to your response next to each statement in Set B.

SET A

a. Independent variable cannot be manipulated
b. Ethical constraints on manipulation
c. Practical constraints on manipulation
d. No constraints on manipulation

SET B   **RESPONSES**

1. Does the use of certain tampons cause toxic shock syndrome?   _____

2. Does heroin addiction among mothers affect Apgar scores of infants?   _____

3. Is the age of a hemodialysis patient related to the incidence of the disequilibrium syndrome?   _____

4. What body positions aid respiratory function?   _____

5. Does the ingestion of saccharin cause cancer in humans?   _____

6. Does a nurse's attitude toward the elderly affect his or her choice of a clinical specialty?   _____

7. Does the use of touch by nursing staff affect patient morale?   _____

8. Does a nurse's gender affect his or her salary and rate of promotion?   _____

9. Does extreme athletic exertion in young women cause amenorrhea?   _____

10. Does assertiveness training affect a psychiatric nurse's
job performance?   _____

■ B. Completion Exercises

Write the words or phrases that correctly complete the sentences below.

1. Researchers generally design their studies to include one or more type of
_____ to make their results more interpretable.

2. In an experiment, the researcher manipulates the _____
variable.

3. The manipulation that the researcher introduces is referred to as the experimental _____.

4. Randomization is performed so that groups will be formed without
_____.

5. Another term for randomization is _____.

6. When data are gathered before the institution of a treatment, the initial
data gathering is referred to as the _____.

7. When more than one independent variable is being simultaneously manipulated by the researcher, the design is referred to as a(n) _____
_____.

8. Each factor in an experimental design must have two or more _____
_____.

9. When neither the subjects nor the individuals collecting data know in
which group a subject is participating, the procedures are called _____
_____.

10. Subjects serve as their own controls in a(n) _____
design.

11. A primary objective of a true experiment is to enable the researcher to
infer _____.

12. When a true experimental design is not used, the control group is usually
referred to as the _____ group.

13. A research design that involves manipulation but lacks the controls of a
quasi-experiment is referred to as a(n) _____
design.

14. A quasi-experimental design that involves repeated observations over time is referred to as a _____ design.

15. The difficulty with a nonequivalent control group design is that the experimental and comparison groups cannot be assumed to be _____ _____ before the intervention.

16. When no variable is manipulated in a study, the research is called _____ _____.

17. Ex post facto research is also referred to as _____ research.

18. In ex post facto research, the investigator does not have control over the _____ variable.

19. Correlation does not prove _____.

20. A prospective design is more rigorous in elucidating casual relationships than a(n) _____ design.

21. A retrospective design that involves a comparison of a group with a specified disease or condition with another group without the disease or condition is called a(n) _____ design.

22. When data are collected at more than one point in time, the design is referred to as _____.

23. Longitudinal studies conducted to determine the long-term outcome of some condition or intervention are called _____ _____.

24. The type of study that collects extensive self-report information on people's attitudes, actions, beliefs, and intentions is called _____ _____.

25. The effectiveness of a policy or program is studied in a(n) _____ _____.

26. The environment should be controlled by the researcher insofar as possible by maximizing _____ in the research conditions.

27. The specifications of an experimental treatment are often referred to as the _____.

28. Using the principle of homogeneity to control extraneous variables is easy but limits the _____ of the findings.

29. Control over extraneous variables is required for the _____ _____ validity of the study.

30. The most persistent threat to the internal validity of studies arises from preexisting differences between groups, or the _____ _____ threat.

31. Changes that occur as the result of time passing rather than as a result of the treatment represent the threat of _____.

32. Events concurrent with the institution of a treatment that can affect the dependent variable constitute the threat of _____.

33. An inadequate sampling plan can affect the _____ validity of a study.

■ C. Study Questions

1. Define the following terms. Compare your definition with the definition in the glossary or in Chapter 8 of the textbook.

   a. Research design _____

   _____

   b. Extraneous variable _____

   _____

   c. Experiment _____

   _____

   d. Manipulation _____

   _____

   e. Randomization _____

   _____

   f. Control group _____

   _____

   g. Clinical trial _____

   _____

   h. Hawthorne effect _____

   _____

   i. Quasi-experiment _____

   _____

   j. Rival hypothesis _____

    _____

   k. Ex post facto research _____

    _____

   l. Retrospective study _____

    _____

  m. Prospective study _____

    _____

   n. Cross-sectional study _____

    _____

   o. Self-selection _____

    _____

   p. Survey research _____

    _____

   q. Outcomes research _____

    _____

   r. Meta-analysis _____

    _____

   s. Matching _____

    _____

   t. Internal validity _____

    _____

   u. Attrition _____

    _____

   v. External validity _____

    _____

2. A nurse researcher found a relationship between teenagers' level of knowledge about birth control and their level of sexual activity. That is, teenagers with higher levels of sexual activity knew more about birth control than teenagers with less sexual activity. Suggest at least three interpretations for this finding.

a. _____

_____

b. _____

_____

c. _____

_____

Does this research situation involve research problem that is *inherently* nonexperimental? Why or why not?

3. Indicate which of the following variables *inherently* can or cannot be manipulated by a researcher.*

a. Age at onset of obesity _____

_____

b. Amount of auditory stimulation _____

_____

c. Number of cigarettes smoked _____

_____

d. Infant's birthweight _____

_____

e. Blood type _____

_____

f. Preoperative anxiety _____

_____

g. Type of nursing curriculum _____

_____

h. Attitudes toward nurses' extended role _____

_____

i. Nurses' shift assignments _____

_____

_____

*Remember that *manipulation* does not refer to whether the variable can be *affected* by a researcher; it refers to the researcher's ability to randomly assign individuals to different levels of the variable or to different groups.

j. Type of birth control method used _____

_____

k. Mother–infant bonding _____

_____

l. Use of atrioventricular shunt versus atrioventricular fistula _____

_____

m. Fluid intake _____

_____

n. Morale of dying patients' family members _____

_____

o. Nurses' fringe benefits _____

_____

4. Refer to the ten hypotheses in Exercises **C.4 and C.5 of Chapter 5 (pages 47–48)**. Indicate below whether these hypotheses could be tested using an experimental/quasi-experimental approach, a nonexperimental approach, or both.

	EXPERIMENTAL/QUASI-EXPERIMENTAL	NONEXPERIMENTAL	BOTH
5a			
5b			
5c			
5d			
5e			
6a			
6b			
6c			
6d			
6e			

5. In the following study, the researchers conducted a double-blind experiment. Review the design for this study and comment on the appropriateness of the double-blind procedures. What biases were the researchers trying to avoid? Were they successful?

Simms, S. G., Rhodes, V. A., & Madsen, R. W. (1993). Comparison of prochlorperazine and lorazepam antiemetic regimens in the control of postchemotherapy symptoms. *Nursing Research, 42,* 234–239.

_____

_____

_____

_____

_____

6. Suppose you wanted to study the coping strategies of AIDS patients at different points in the progress of the disease. Design a cross-sectional study to research this question, describing how subjects would be selected. Now design a longitudinal study to research the same problem. Identify the strengths and weaknesses of the two approaches.

_____

_____

_____

_____

_____

7. Suppose that you were interested in testing the hypothesis that the use of IUDs could cause infertility. Describe how such a hypothesis could be tested using a retrospective design. Now describe a prospective design for the same study. Compare the strengths and weaknesses of the two approaches.

_____

_____

_____

_____

_____

8. Suppose that you are studying the effects of range-of-motion exercises on radical mastectomy patients. You start your experiment with 50 experimental subjects and 50 control subjects. Your intervention requires the experimental subjects to come for daily sessions over a two-week period, while control subjects come only once at the end of two weeks. Your final group sizes are 40 for the experimental group and 49 for the control group. The results of your study indicate that the experimental group did

better in raising the arm of the affected side above head level. What effects, if any, do you think the subject attrition might have on the internal validity of your study?

_____

_____

_____

_____

_____

9. Below are several research problems. Indicate for each whether you think the problem should be studied using a survey approach or using an in-depth qualitative approach. Justify your response.

   a. By what process do new nursing home residents learn to adapt to their environments? _____

_____

_____

   b. To what extent are dietary habits and exercise patterns in healthy adults related? _____

_____

_____

   c. What is the relationship between a teenager's health-risk appraisal and various forms of risk-taking behavior (e.g., smoking, unsafe sex)? _____

_____

_____

   d. What aspects of the lifestyles of urban disadvantaged women place them at especially high risk for pregnancy and childbirth complications? _____

_____

_____

   e. How do older men adjust to problems of sexual functioning? _____

_____

_____

■ D. Application Exercises

1. Below is a brief description of the research design for a fictitious study, followed by a critique. Do you agree with the critique. Can you add other comments relevant to the design of this study? (Box 8-1 offers some guiding questions.)

Fictitious Study. Bikowicz (2001) hypothesized that nursing effectiveness is higher in primary nursing than in team nursing. To test this hypothesis, she obtained data based on the nursing care of 100 patients in two medical-surgical units at the Wilton Hospital (which used primary nursing) and data from a similar sample of patients hospitalized at Ballston Hospital (which used team nursing). In both cases, the nursing approach was one that had been in place for more than five years. Bikowicz used three measures of nursing effectiveness: patient's length of stay in hospital, ratings of effectiveness by an objective expert observer, and total number of errors of omission and commission by the nursing staff. Bikowicz realized that numerous factors influence nursing effectiveness and that these factors needed to be controlled to test the research hypothesis. However, random assignment of nurses to the two types of nursing and random assignment of patients to hospitals was not possible. Therefore, Bikowicz took other steps to enhance the internal validity of the study. First, she designed her study in such a way that the conditions in the two hospitals were as comparable as possible. For example, she selected two private hospitals that were similar in size, modernity, reputation, nurses' pay scale, and proximity to an urban center. She focused on two medical-surgical units that were similar with respect to staff-patient ratio, number of beds, type of medical problems, and number of private and semiprivate rooms.

Bikowicz also recognized that staff characteristics were important. Therefore, a group of 25 nurses in each hospital who provided the care during the study were matched with respect to number of years of nursing experience (more than five years or fewer than five years) and educational credentials (baccalaureate degree or not). Finally, the 100 patients in each hospital were matched in terms of their gender and age (in five-year groupings).

The data were collected by two objective observers who had no affiliation with either of the two hospitals and no personal acquaintance with any of the nursing staff or patients. The data supported

Bikowicz's hypothesis that primary nursing is more effective than team nursing.

Critique. Bikowicz was interested in elucidating a causal relationship between type of nursing and nursing effectiveness; in essence, she was performing an evaluation of nursing approach. Given this aim, her decision to design a tightly controlled study seems well-advised, particularly given the nonexperimental nature of the study. Bikowicz had no control over the implementation of either the primary or the team nursing. She tested her hypothesis using intact, preestablished groups of nurses and their patients. Although Bikowicz had to work with existing conditions, she nevertheless was careful in designing a study that controlled for numerous external and intrinsic extraneous variables. She maintained constancy over numerous external conditions, such as the hospital settings and the data collection procedures.

Bikowicz controlled several important intrinsic characteristics (of both nurses and patients) through matching. Although this procedure has numerous shortcomings, the use of matching was in this case preferable to totally ignoring the problem of extraneous variables. One alternative would have been to use the principle of homogeneity (e.g., use all baccalaureate nurses with more than five years of experience, or use patients in a similar age range), but this would have seriously limited the generalizability of the results. The problem with matching, as noted earlier, is that only two or three matching variables can be used, and there may be far more than two or three extraneous variables. For example, such factors as a nurse's age, amount of continuing education, level of empathy, and attitudes toward type of nursing approach presumably affect type of nursing effectiveness. If systematic differences in these variables existed between nurses in the two hospitals (or if there were other important differences between the two groups of patients), then such differences represent rival explanations, competing with the type of nursing approach as causes of the differences of the ratings of nursing effectiveness. Thus, selection is the primary threat to the internal validity of this study. If some external event affecting nursing performance occurred in one or both hospitals during the data collection period, then history might also have been a threat.

In summary, the researcher took many commendable steps to control extraneous variables in the study. Given the constraints of not being able to manipulate the independent variable (i.e., random-ize nurses and patients to groups or randomize hospitals to type of nursing approach), matching was one of the best alternatives to con-trolling extraneous variables. The only more rigorous approach would have been to gather data on any other extraneous variables (e.g., nurses' ages or amounts of continuing education) and to con-trol these variables statistically using analysis of covariance. It might be noted that Bikowicz might have strengthened her conclusions re-garding the effectiveness of primary versus team nursing if she also had undertaken an in-depth qualitative study of the nursing care of typical patients in both hospitals.

2. Below is a brief description of the research design for a fictitious study. Read the summary and then respond to the questions that follow.

Seligman and Jolly (2001) wanted to test the effectiveness of a new relaxation/biofeedback intervention on menopause symptoms. They invited women who presented themselves in an outpatient clinic with complaints of severe hot flashes to participate in the study of the experimental treatment. These 30 women were asked to record, every day for one week before their treatment, the frequency and duration of their hot flashes. During the intervention, which in-volved six one-hour sessions over a three-week period, the women again recorded their symptoms. Then, four weeks after the treat-ment, the women were asked to record their hot flashes over a five-day period. At the end of the study, Seligman and Jolly found that both the frequency and average duration of the hot flashes had been significantly reduced in this sample of women. They concluded that their new treatment was an effective alternative to estrogen replace-ment therapy in treating menopausal hot flashes.

Review and critique this study. Suggest alternative designs for testing the effectiveness of the treatment. To assist you in your critique, here are some guiding questions:
   a. What are the independent and dependent variables in this study?
   b. Is the design described above experimental, quasi-experimental, or pre-experimental?
   c. The investigators concluded that the outcome (i.e., the reduction in the frequency and duration of the women's hot flashes) was attributable to the experimental treatment. Can you offer one or more alternative ex-planations to account for the outcome? Discuss the inference of causal-ity in the context of this research design.

   d. Consider your responses to part c above. If you have identified any weaknesses in the design of this research, suggest a modified design that would improve the study. In what way does your new design eliminate the problems of the original design?

3. Below are several suggested research articles. Read one or more of these articles, and respond to questions a through d from Question D.2 in terms of these actual research studies.

   ■ Christman, S. K., Fish, A. F., Bernhard, L., Frid, D. J., Smith, B. A., & Mitchell, G. L. (2000). Continuous handrail support, oxygen uptake, and heart rate in women during submaximal step treadmill exercise. *Research in Nursing & Health, 23,* 35–42.

   ■ DeFloor, T. (2000). The effect of position and mattress on interface pressure. *Applied Nursing Research, 13,* 2–11.

   ■ Hill, A. S., Kurkowski, T. B., & Garcia, J. (2000). Oral support measures used in feeding the preterm infant. *Nursing Research, 49,* 2–10.

   ■ McCurren, C., Dowe, D., Rattle, D., & Looney, S. (1999). Depression among nursing home elders. *Applied Nursing Research, 12,* 185–195.

   ■ Varda, K. E., & Behnke, R. S. (2000). The effect of timing of initial bath on newborn's temperature. *Journal of Obstetric, Gynecologic, and Neonatal Nursing, 29,* 27–32.

4. Another brief summary of the research design for a fictitious study is presented next. Read the summary and then answer the questions that follow.

Reynolds (2000) hypothesized that the absence of socioemotional supports among the elderly results in a high level of chronic health problems and low morale. She tested this hypothesis by interviewing a sample of 250 residents of one community who were aged 65 years and older. The respondents were randomly selected from a list of town residents. Reynolds used several measures regarding the availability of socioemotional supports: (1) whether the respondent lived with any kin; (2) whether the respondent had any living children who resided within 30 minutes away; (3) the total number of interactions the respondent had had in the previous week with kin not residing in his or her household; and (4) the number of close friends in whom the respondent felt he or she could confide. Based on responses to the various questions on social support, respondents were classified in one of three groups: low social support, moderate social support, and high social support.

In a six-month follow-up interview, Reynolds collected information from 214 respondents about the frequency and intensity of the respondents' illnesses in the preceding six months, their hospitalization record, their overall satisfaction with life, and their attitudes toward their own aging. An analysis of the data revealed that the low-support group had significantly more health problems, lower life satisfaction ratings, and lower acceptance of their aging than the other two groups. Reynolds concluded that the availability of social supports resulted in better physical and mental adjustment to old age.

Review and critique this study. Suggest alternative designs for testing the researcher's hypothesis. To assist you in your critique, here are some guiding questions:

a. What are the independent and dependent variables in this study?
b. Is this research nonexperimental? If so, is it *inherently* nonexperimental? Why or why not? If so, what *type* of nonexperimental research is it?
c. Examine the criteria for causality presented in Chapter 8 of the text. Does this study meet all the criteria for establishing causality?
d. The researcher concluded that her independent variable "caused" certain outcomes. Can you offer two or more alternative explanations to account for the outcome?
e. Consider your responses to parts b and c above. If you have identified any weaknesses in the design of this research, suggest modifications that would improve the study design.

5. Below are several suggested research articles. Read the introductory and methods sections of one or more of these articles, and respond to questions a through e from Question D.4 in terms of these actual research studies.

■ Anderson, B., Higgins, L., & Rozmus, C. (2000). Critical pathways: Application to selected patient outcomes following coronary artery bypass graft. *Applied Nursing Research, 12,* 168–174.

■ Anderson, M. A., Helms, L. B., Hanson, K. S., & DeVilder, N. W. (1999). Unplanned hospital readmissions: A home care perspective. *Nursing Research, 48,* 299–307.

■ Connelly, C. D. (1998). Hopefulness, self-esteem, and perceived social support among pregnant and nonpregnant adolescents. *Western Journal of Nursing Research, 20,* 195–209.

■ Gibson, P. R., Cheavens, J., & Warren, M. L. (1998). Social support in persons with self-reported sensitivity to chemicals. *Research in Nursing & Health, 21,* 103–115.

■ Youngblut, J. M., Madigan, E. A., Neff, D. F., Deoisres, W., Siripul, P., & Brooten, D. (2000). Employment patterns and timing of birth in women with high-risk pregnancies. *Journal of Obstetric, Gynecologic, and Neonatal Nursing, 29,* 137–144.

6. Another brief summary of the research design for a fictitious study is presented next. Read the summary and then answer the questions that follow.

Butcher (2001) studied the contraceptive practices of university students at three large Midwestern universities. In addition to obtaining descriptive information, he wanted to test the hypothesis that students who report favorable experiences with health care personnel relating to contraceptives are more likely than those with unfavorable experiences to practice birth control effectively. A random sample of 500 students from each university was sent a mailed questionnaire. A total of 715 usable questionnaires were returned.

The questionnaire included questions on sexual experience, contraceptive use history, perceived ease of access to birth control, feelings about seeking out contraceptive information, knowledge of on-campus contraceptive services, and experiences with health care personnel related to contraceptives. The questionnaire also asked about the student's age, ethnicity, year in college, major, father's occupation, marital status, religion, and grade point average.

Butcher's data revealed that while most students were sexually experienced, fewer than half had used any birth control during their last intercourse. About 60 percent of the sexually active students had had a contact with health care personnel relating to contraceptives, and of these, 70 percent described their experience in positive terms. In comparing those who had had favorable and unfavorable experiences, Butcher found that a significantly higher percentage of those with a favorable experience (68% versus 42%) had used some form of contraceptive at last intercourse. He concluded that a favorable experience with health care personnel leads to better contraceptive utilization. He speculated that those with more positive experiences were better informed about and more accepting of contraception than those with negative experiences and hence practiced birth control more conscientiously.

Review and critique this study. Suggest alternative methods for conducting this research. To assist you in your critique, here are some guiding questions:

a. What are the independent and dependent variables in this study?

b. Is this research nonexperimental? If so, is it *inherently* nonexperimental? Why or why not?

c. What type of research study is this, in terms of the types discussed in this chapter? Could the same research problem be studied using an alternative approach (i.e., one of the other types of research discussed in the chapter)?

d. Examine the criteria for causality presented in Chapter 8 of the text. Does this study meet all the criteria for establishing causality?

e. The researcher concluded that the independent variable "caused" a certain outcome. Can you offer alternative explanations to account for the outcome?

f. Consider your responses to parts b and c, above. If you have identified any weaknesses in the design of this research, suggest modifications that would improve the study design.

7. Below are several suggested research articles. Skim one or more of these articles and respond to questions a through f from Question D.6 in terms of this actual research study.

■ Greif, J., Hewitt, W., & Armstrong, M. L. (1999). Tattooing and body piercing. *Clinical Nursing Research, 8,* 368–385.

■ Hall, L. A., Sachs, B., & Rayens, M. K. (1998). Mothers' potential for child abuse: The roles of childhood abuse and social resources. *Nursing Research, 47,* 87–95.

■ Keane, A., Brennan, A. W., & Picket, M. (2000). A typology of residential fire survivors' multidimensional needs. *Western Journal of Nursing Research, 22,* 263–284.

■ McCorkle, R. et al. (1998). The effects of home nursing care for patients during terminal illness on the bereaved's psychological distress. *Nursing Research, 47,* 2–10.

■ Oka, M., & Chaboyer, W. (1999). Dietary behaviors and sources of support in hemodialysis patients. *Clinical Nursing Research, 8,* 302–317.

■ E. Special Projects

1. Suppose that you were interested in testing the hypothesis that a regular regimen of exercise reduces blood pressure, improves cardiovascular efficiency, and increases coronary circulation. Design a quasi-experiment to test the hypothesis. Evaluate this design in terms of the ability to make

causal inferences. Design a true experiment to test the same hypothesis and compare the kinds of conclusions that can be drawn with this design with those from the quasi-experiment. Describe how you might design an ex post facto study to test the same hypothesis. What are the most salient threats to the internal validity of the designs?

2. Suppose that you were interested in testing the hypothesis that the use of oral contraceptives causes breast cancer. Describe how such a hypothesis could be tested using a retrospective design. Now describe a prospective design for the same study. Compare the strengths and weaknesses of the two approaches. Could an experimental or quasi-experimental design be used? Why or why not?

3. Suppose that you wanted to compare premature and normal babies in terms of their development at 5 years of age. Describe how you would design such a study, being careful to indicate what extraneous variables you would need to control and how you would control them. Identify the major threats to the internal validity of your design.

4. A nurse researcher is interested in testing the effect of a special high fiber diet on cardiovascular risk factors (e.g., cholesterol level) in adults with a family history of cardiovascular disease. Describe a design you would recommend for this problem, being careful to indicate what extraneous variables you would need to control and how you would control them. Identify the major threats to the internal validity of your design.

CHAPTER 9

Understanding Qualitative Research Design

■ A. Matching Exercises

1. Match each descriptive statement from Set B with one of the research traditions from Set A. Indicate the letter corresponding to your response next to each item in Set B.

SET A

a. Ethnography
b. Phenomenology
c. Grounded theory
d. Ethnography, phenomenology, and grounded theory

SET B   RESPONSES

1. Is rooted in a philosophical tradition developed by Husserl and Heidegger. _____

2. Studies both broadly defined cultures and more narrowly defined ones. _____

3. Uses qualitative data to address questions of interest. _____

4. Is an approach to the study of social processes and social structures. _____

5. Is concerned with the lived experiences of humans. _____

6. Strives to achieve an emic perspective on the members of a group. _____

7. Is closely related to a research tradition called hermeneutics. _____

8. Uses a procedure referred to as constant comparison. _____

9. Stems from a discipline other than nursing. _____

10. Developed by the sociologists Glaser and Strauss. _____

2. Match each descriptive statement from Set B with one of the statements from Set A. Indicate the letter corresponding to your response next to each item in Set B.

SET A

a. Qualitative data

b. Quantitative data

c. Both qualitative and quantitative data

d. Neither qualitative nor quantitative data

SET B   **RESPONSES**

1. Should be collected to help improve nursing practice.   _____

2. Are especially useful for understanding dynamic processes.   _____

3. Are often collected in large-scale surveys.   _____

4. Are useful in *proving* the validity of theories.   _____

5. Are usually collected by phenomenological researchers.   _____

6. Can profit from triangulation.   _____

7. Are often used in tests of causal relationships.   _____

8. Can contribute to theoretical insights.   _____

9. Require validity checks.   _____

10. Tend to be collected from small samples.   _____

■ B. Completion Exercises

Write the words or phrases that correctly complete the sentences below.

1. The design for a qualitative study is often called a(n) _____ _____ design.

2. Qualitative researchers are often adept at performing many diverse tasks and are sometimes referred to as _____.

3. The disciplinary roots of ethnography is _____; of ethology, _____; and of ethnomethodology, _____

4. Ethnographic research focuses on human _____.

5. An ethnographic study of a Peruvian village would be called a _____ _____, while an ethnographic study of a ward in a psychiatric hospital would be called a _____.

6. The concept of _____ is frequently used by ethnographers to describe the significant role of the researcher in interpreting a culture.

7. Phenomenologic research focuses on the _____ of phenomena as experienced by people.

8. Phenomenologists study the various aspects of the lived experience including lived space or _____; lived body or _____; lived time or _____; or lived human relations or _____.

9. The primary purpose of _____ is to generate comprehensive explanations of phenomena that are grounded in reality.

10. In a grounded theory study, the technique referred to as _____ _____ is used to compare new data with previously collected data to identify commonalities and refine categories.

11. Qualitative and quantitative data may, for some research problems, be _____ in that they "mutually supply each other's lack."

12. The major conceptual frameworks of nursing demand neither _____ nor _____ data.

13. Progress in a developing area of research tends to be _____ _____ and can profit from multiple feedback loops.

14. A major advantage of integrating different approaches is potential enhancements to the study's _____.

15. A frequent application of multimethod studies is in the development of research _____.

16. In a quantitative study, the inclusion of qualitative data might facilitate the _____ of the findings, and vice versa.

■ C. Study Questions

1. Define the following terms. Use the textbook to compare your definition with the definition in Chapter 9 or in the Glossary.

a. Bricolage _____

_____

b. Discourse analysis _____

_____

c. Hermeneutics _____

_____

d. Symbolic interaction _____

_____

e. Emic perspective _____

_____

f. Etic perspective _____

_____

g. Ethnonursing research _____

_____

h. Descriptive phenomenology _____

_____

i. Interpretive phenomenology _____

_____

j. Being-in-the-world _____

_____

k. Bracketing _____

_____

l. Multimethod research _____

_____

m. Black box _____

_____

n. Complementarity _____

_____

2. For each of the research questions below, indicate what type of qualitative research tradition would likely guide the inquiry.

   a. What is the social psychological process experienced by couples experiencing infertility? _____

   _____

   b. How does the culture of a suicide survivors self-help group contribute to the grieving process? _____

   _____

   c. What are the power dynamics that arise in conversations between nurses and bed-ridden nursing home patients? _____

   _____

   d. What is the lived experience of the spousal caretaker of an Alzheimer patient? _____

   _____

3. Read the following two studies, which exemplify ethnographic and phenomenological studies. What were the central phenomena under investigation? Compare and contrast the methods used in these two studies (e.g., How were data collected? How many study participants were there? To what extent did the design unfold while the researchers were in the field?).

   ■ *Ethnographic Study:* Eastland, L. S. (1995). Recovery as an interactive process: Explanation and empowerment in 12-step programs. *Qualitative Health Research, 5*, 292–314.

   ■ *Phenomenological Study:* Chase, S. K., Melloni, M., & Savage, A. (1997). A forever healing: The lived experience of venous ulcer disease. *Journal of Vascular Nursing, 15*, 73–78.

   _____

   _____

   _____

   _____

   _____

4. Read one of the following studies, in which qualitative data were gathered and analyzed to address a research question. Suggest ways in which the collection of quantitative data might have enriched the study, strengthened its validity, and/or enhanced its interpretability. (Alternatively, defend the collection of qualitative data exclusively.)

   ■ Dickson, G. (2000). Aboriginal grandmothers' experience with health promotion and participatory action research. *Qualitative Health Research, 10,* 188–213.

   ■ Herth, K. (1998). Integrating hearing loss into one's life. *Qualitative Health Research, 8,* 207–223.

   ■ Kuyper, M. B., & Wester, F. (1998). In the shadow: The impact of chronic illness on the patient's partner. *Qualitative Health Research, 8,* 237–253.

   ■ Niska, K. J., Lia-Hoagberg, B., & Snyder, M. (1997). Parental concerns of Mexican American first-time mothers and fathers. *Public Health Nursing, 14,* 111–117.

   ■ Radwin, L. (2000). Oncology patients' perceptions of quality nursing care. *Research in Nursing & Health, 23,* 179–190.

   _____

   _____

   _____

   _____

   _____

5. Read one of the following studies, in which quantitative data were gathered and analyzed to address a research question. Suggest ways in which the collection of qualitative data might have enriched the study, strengthened its validity, or enhanced its interpretability:

   ■ Bull, M. J., Hansen, H. E., & Gross, C. R. (2000). Differences in family caregiver outcomes by their level of involvement in discharge planning. *Applied Nursing Research, 13,* 76–82.

   ■ Jadack, R. A., Pare, B., Kachur, S. P., & Zenilman, J. M. (2000). Self-reported weapon ownership, use, and violence experience among clients accessing an inner-city sexually transmitted disease clinic. *Research in Nursing & Health, 23,* 213–221.

   ■ Lee, H., Kohlman, G., Lee, K., & Schiller, N. B. (2000). Fatigue, mood, and hemodynamic patterns after myocardial infarction. *Applied Nursing Research, 13,* 60–69.

■ Meisenhelder, J. B., & Chandler, E. N. (2000). Faith, prayer, and health outcomes in elderly Native Americans. *Clinical Nursing Research*, 9, 191–203.

■ Milne, J. (2000). The impact of information on health behaviors of older adults with urinary incontinence. *Clinical Nursing Research*, 9, 161–176.

■ D. Application Exercises

1. Below is a brief description of an integrated qualitative-quantitative study, followed by a critique. Do you agree with this critique? Can you add other comments regarding this study design? (Box 9-1 offers some guiding questions.)

   Fictitious Study. Borel (2001) conducted a study designed to examine the emotional well-being of women who had had a mastectomy. Borel wanted to develop an in-depth understanding of the emotional experiences of women as they recovered from their surgery, including the process by which they handled their fears, their concerns about their sexuality, their levels of anxiety and depression, their methods of coping, and their social supports.

   Borel's basic study design was a field study, loosely within a grounded theory tradition. She gathered information from a sample of 25 women, primarily by means of in-depth interviews with the women on two occasions. The first interviews were scheduled within one month after the surgery. Follow-up interviews were conducted about twelve months after the surgery. Several of the women in the sample participated in a support group, and Borel attended and made observations at several of those meetings. Additionally, Borel decided to interview the "significant other" (usually the women's husbands) of most of the women, when she learned that the women's emotional well-being was linked to the manner in which the significant other was reacting to the surgery.

In addition to the rich, in-depth information she gathered, Borel wanted to be able to better interpret the emotional status of the women. Therefore, at both the original and follow-up interview with the women, she administered a psychological scale known as the Center for Epidemiological Studies Depression Scale (CES-D), a quantitative measure that has scores that can range from 0 to 60. This scale has been widely used in community populations, and has cut-off scores designating when a person is at risk of clinical depression (i.e., a score of 16 and above).

Borel's qualitative analysis showed that the basic process underlying psychological recovery from the mastectomy was something she labeled "Gaining by Losing," a process that involved heightened self-awareness and self-respect after an initial period of despair and self-pity. The process also involved, for some, a strengthening of personal relationships with significant others, whereas for others, it resulted in the birth of awareness of fundamental deficiencies in their relationships. The quantitative findings confirmed that a very high percentage of women were at risk of being depressed at one month after the mastectomy, but at twelve months, levels of depression were actually modestly lower than in the general population of women.

Critique. In her study, Borel embedded a quantitative measure into the field work in an interesting manner. The bulk of data were qualitative—in-depth interviews and in-depth observations. However, she also opted to include a well-known measure of depression, which provided her with an important context for interpreting her data. A major advantage of using the CES-D (aside from the fact that the CES-D has a good reputation) is that this scale has known characteristics in the general population, and therefore provided a built-in "comparison group."

Borel used a flexible design that allowed her to use her initial data to guide her inquiry. For example, she decided to conduct in-depth interviews with significant others when she learned their importance to the women's process of emotional recovery. Borel did do some advance planning, however, that provided loose guidance. For example, although her questioning undoubtedly evolved while in the field, she had the foresight to realize that to capture a process, she would need to collect data longitudinally. She also made the up-front decision to use the CES-D to supplement the in-depth interviews.

In this study, the findings from the qualitative and quantitative portions of the study were complementary. Both portions of the study confirmed that the women initially had emotional "losses," but eventually they recovered and "gained" in terms of their emotional well-being and their self-awareness. This example illustrates how the validity of study findings can be enhanced by the blending of qualitative and quantitative data. If the qualitative data alone had been gathered, Borel might not have gotten a good handle on the degree to which the women had actually "recovered" (vis à vis women who had never had a mastectomy). Conversely, if she had collected only the CES-D data, she would have had no insights into the process by which the recovery occurred.

2. Below is a brief description of a fictitious qualitative study. Read the summary and then respond to the questions that follow.

Dake and Talman (2000) investigated women who had given their babies up for adoption. They conducted a grounded theory study to examine the process women go through during the first year after they have relinquished their babies. Dake and Talman obtained their sample of 28 women through a local support group for women who had given their babies up for adoption. All 28 participants were white, middle/upper-middle class women, ranging in age from 18 to 44. Some of the women (8) were married, but most (20) were single or divorced. The majority of women (18) had no other children, but ten were mothers with other children at home. Twelve women had made their decision regarding adoption during the first trimester of their pregnancy. Ten women did not decide until their third trimester, and the remaining six women were still struggling with their decision in the hospital after they had delivered their babies. Each of the 28 participants was interviewed once in depth and asked about her post-birth experience. Interviews, which were tape recorded, ranged in length from 30 to 60 minutes. When all 28 interviews were completed, the constant comparative method was used to analyze the data. Analysis of the transcribed interviews revealed that the basic problem these women had to cope with over the first year after relinquishing their newborns was mourning the child they would never have. Dake and Talman reported that four themes emerged from the data analysis that captured the experience of the participants. These four themes were:

1. Guilt consumed the women over their giving their babies up for adoption.
2. Women grieved the loss of their children they would never have to love and watch grow up.
3. The women were still immersed in agonizing questioning over whether their decision to relinquish their baby was the right one.
4. The women had not yet fully come to terms with their choice.

Review and critique this study. Suggest alternative data collection and analysis approaches. To assist you in your critique, here are some guiding questions.

a. How structured or flexible was the research design in this study? Comment on how the degree of structure benefitted or detracted from the study.
b. Was this study squarely within one single qualitative tradition? Identify the tradition(s).
c. Was the use of a qualitative approach justified, given the researcher's aims? Would a quantitative approach have been appropriate?

3. Below are several suggested research articles of qualitative studies. Read one or more of these articles and respond to parts **a** to **c** of Question D.2 in terms of these actual research studies.

   ■ Draucker, C. B., & Stern, P. N. (2000). Women's responses to sexual violence by male intimates. *Western Journal of Nursing Research, 22* 385–406.

   ■ Felten, B. S. (2000). Resilience in a multicultural sample of community-dwelling women older than age 85. *Clinical Nursing Research, 9,* 102–123,

   ■ Hall, B.A. (1998). Patterns of spirituality in persons with advanced HIV disease. *Research in Nursing & Health, 21,* 143–153.

   ■ Hilton, B. A., Crawford, J. A., & Tarko, M. A. (2000). Men's perspectives on individual and family coping with their wives' breast cancer and chemotherapy. *Western Journal of Nursing Research, 22,* 438–459.

   ■ Orne, R. M., Fishman, S. J., Manka, M., & Pagnozzi, M. (2000). Living on the edge: A phenomenological study of medically uninsured working Americans. *Research in Nursing & Health, 23,* 204–212.

   ■ Shidler, S. (1998). A systemic perspective of life-prolonging treatment decision making. *Qualitative Health Research, 8,* 254–269.

4. Below is a summary of a fictitious multimethod study. Read the summary and then respond to the questions that follow.

Zack (2000) conducted a study to investigate breastfeeding practices among teenaged mothers, who have been found in many studies to be less likely than older mothers to breastfeed. Using birth records from two large hospitals, Zack contacted 250 young women between 15 and 19 years of age who had given birth in the previous year and invited them to participate in a survey. Those who agreed to participate ($N = 185$) were interviewed by telephone (when possible), using a structured interview that asked about breastfeeding practices, attitudes toward motherhood, availability of social supports, and conflicting demands, such as school attendance or employment. Several psychological scales (including measures of depression and self-esteem) were also administered. Teenagers without a telephone were interviewed in person in their own homes. All the teenagers interviewed at home were also interviewed in greater depth, using a topic guide that focused on such areas as feelings about breastfeeding, the decision-making process that led them to decide whether to breastfeed, barriers to breastfeeding, and intentions to breastfeed with any subsequent children. Zack used the quantitative data to determine the characteristics associated with breastfeeding status and duration. The qualitative data were used to interpret and validate the quantitative findings.

Review and critique this study. Suggest alternative data collection and analysis approaches. To assist you in your critique, here are some guiding questions:

   a. Which of the aims of integration, if any, were served by this study?
   b. What was the researcher's basic strategy for integration? How effective was this strategy in addressing the aims of integration?
   c. Suggest ways of altering the design of the study and the data collection approach to further promote integrative aims.
   d. Would the study have been stronger if it had involved the collection of quantitative data only? Qualitative data only? Why or why not?

5. Below are several suggested research articles of studies that used an integrated approach. Read one or more of these articles and respond to questions **a** through **d** from Question D.4 in terms of these actual research studies.

- Courts, N. F. (2000). Psychosocial adjustment of patients on home hemodialysis and their dialysis partners. *Clinical Nursing Research, 9,* 177–190.

- Im, E. & Meleis, A. I. (2000). Meanings of menopause to Korean immigrant women. *Western Journal of Nursing Research, 22,* 84–102.

- McDonald, D. D., McNulty, J., Erickson, K., & Weiskopf, C. (2000). Communicating pain and pain management needs after surgery. *Applied Nursing Research, 13,* 70–75.

- Melillo, K. D., Williamson, E., Futrell, M., & Chamberlain, C. (1997). A self-assessment tool to measure older adults' perceptions regarding physical fitness and exercise activity. *Journal of Advanced Nursing, 25,* 1220–1226.

- Smith, C. E. et al. (1998). Continuous positive airway pressure: Patients' and caregivers' learning needs and barriers to use. *Heart & Lung, 27,* 99–108.

■ E. Special Projects

1. Prepare a research question that could be investigated within each of the following qualitative traditions:

a. Ethnographic research: _____

_____

b. Phenomenological research: _____

_____

c. Grounded theory: _____

_____

2. Prepare two problem statements that would be amenable to multimethod research.

_____

_____

_____

_____

_____

CHAPTER 10

Examining Sampling Plans

■ A. Matching Exercises

1. Match each statement relating to sampling for quantitative studies from Set B with one of the phrases from Set A. Indicate the letter corresponding to your response next to each of the statements in Set B.

SET A

a. Probability sampling

b. Nonprobability sampling

c. Both probability and nonprobability sampling

d. Neither probability nor nonprobability sampling

SET B   **RESPONSES**

1. Includes systematic sampling.   _____

2. Allows an estimation of the magnitude of sampling error.   _____

3. Guarantees a representative sample.   _____

4. Includes quota sampling.   _____

5. Yields better results when the samples are large.   _____

6. Elements are selected by nonrandom methods.   _____

7. Can be used with entire populations or with selected strata from the populations.   _____

8. Used to select populations.   _____

9. Provides an equal chance of elements being selected.   _____

10. Is required when the population is completely homogeneous.   _____

2. Match each type of sampling approach from Set B with one of the phrases from Set A. Indicate the letter corresponding to your response next to each of the statements in Set B.

SET A

a. Sampling approach for quantitative studies

b. Sampling approach for qualitative studies

c. Sampling approach for either quantitative or qualitative studies

d. Sampling approach for neither quantitative nor qualitative studies

SET B   **RESPONSES**

1. Typical case sampling   _____

2. Purposive sampling   _____

3. Cluster sampling   _____

4. Maximum variation sampling   _____

5. Extreme/deviant case sampling   _____

6. Snowball sampling   _____

7. Stratified random sampling   _____

8. Quota sampling   _____

9. Power sampling   _____

10. Theoretical sampling   _____

■ B. Completion Exercises

Write the words or phrases that correctly complete the sentences below.

1. A(n)_____ is a subset of the units that comprise the population.

2. The main criterion for evaluating a sample in a quantitative study is its _____ of the population being studied.

3. A sample in a quantitative study would be considered _____ _____ if it systematically overrepresented or underrepresented a segment of the population.

4. If a population is completely _____ with respect to key attributes, then any sample is as good as any other.

5. Another term used for convenience sample is _____ _____.

6. Quota samples are essentially convenience samples from selected _____ of the population.

7. Another term for a purposive sampling in a quantitative context is _____ sampling; in a qualitative context, the terms _____ or _____ sampling are sometimes used for purposive sampling.

8. The most basic type of probability sampling is referred to as _____ .

9. When disproportionate sampling is used, an adjustment procedure known as _____ is normally used to estimate population values.

10. Another term used to refer to cluster sampling is _____ sampling.

11. In systematic samples, the distance between selected elements is referred to as the _____ .

12. Differences between population values and sample values are referred to as _____ .

13. If a quantitative researcher has confidence in his or her sampling design, the results of a study can reasonably be generalized to the _____ population.

14. As the size of a sample _____ , the probability of drawing a deviant sample diminishes.

15. If a researcher wanted to draw a systematic sample of 100 from a population of 3000, the sampling interval would be _____ .

16. In a qualitative study, sampling decisions are often guided by the potential a data source had to be _____ -rich.

17. In _____ sampling, the researcher purposefully selects cases with a wide range of variation on dimensions of interest.

18. _____ sampling involves selecting study participants to highlight the average situation.

■ C. Study Questions

1. Define the following terms. Compare your definition with the definition in Chapter 10 of the textbook or in the glossary.

   a. Sampling _____

b. Probability sampling _____

_____

c. Nonprobability sampling _____

_____

d. Stratum _____

_____

e. Eligibility criteria _____

_____

f. Convenience sample _____

_____

g. Snowball sampling _____

_____

h. Quota sample _____

_____

i. Random sample _____

_____

j. Sampling frame _____

_____

k. Disproportionate sampling design _____

_____

l. Systematic sampling _____

_____

m. Theoretical sampling _____

_____

n. Maximum variation sampling _____

_____

o. Extreme case sampling _____

_____

p. Data saturation _____

_____

2. Identify the type of quantitative sampling design used in the following examples:

   a. One hundred inmates randomly sampled from a random selection of five federal penitentiaries _____

   b. All the nurses participating in a continuing education seminar _____

   _____

   c. Every twentieth patient admitted to the emergency room between January and June _____

   d. The first twenty male and the first twenty female patients admitted to the hospital with hypothermia _____

   e. A sample of 250 members randomly selected from a roster of American Nurses' Association members _____

   f. Twenty-five people whose family members had attempted suicide, most of whom were referred by other people already in the sample

   _____

3. Nurse A is planning to study the effects of maternal stress, maternal depression, maternal age, family economic resources, and social support on a child's socioemotional development among both intact and mother-headed families. Nurse B is planning to study body position on patients' respiratory functioning. Describe the kinds of samples that the two nurses would need to use. Which nurse would need the larger sample? Defend your answer.

   _____

   _____

   _____

   _____

   _____

4. Suppose a researcher in your area were interested in studying the smoking habits of nurses in a survey. Suggest a possible target and accessible population for this study. What strata might be identified by the researcher if a quota or stratified random sample were used?

   _____

   _____

   _____

5. Suppose a qualitative researcher wanted to study the life quality of cancer survivors. Suggest what the researcher might do to obtain a maximum variation sample; a typical case sample; a homogeneous sample; and an extreme case sample.

■ D. Application Exercises

1. Below is a brief description of the sampling plan of a fictitious study, followed by a critique. Do you agree with this critique? Can you add other comments relevant to the sampling plan of this study? (Box 10-1 offers some guiding questions.)

   Fictitious Study. Bao (2000) designed a quantitative study to investigate nurses' attitudes toward surrogate motherhood, test-tube babies, and other nontraditional reproductive options. She defined her target population as all RNs in the United States. She realized, however, that she did not have direct access to the entire population for selecting a sample. Therefore, she specified as her accessible population RNs in the state of Massachusetts. She contacted the directors of nursing in 12 hospitals chosen to represent urban and rural settings and public and private auspices and enlisted their cooperation. She asked these directors to distribute 30 questionnaires to random samples of RNs in the hospitals. The number of completed questionnaires obtained from 10 hospitals (the other two hospitals did not wish to participate) ranged from a low of 16 to a high of 28, for a total of 238 completed questionnaires.

   Critique. The sampling design used by Bao is a multistage design that combines both nonprobability and probability components. Bao handpicked 12 hospitals that yielded, in her judgment, a good mix in terms of locations and auspices. The first stage of the design, therefore, can be described as purposive sampling. Bao could have obtained a listing of all Massachusetts facilities and randomly chosen 12. With such a small sample of hospitals, however, it is conceivable that a skewed sample might have been obtained (e.g., no rural hospitals). If the location and auspices of the hospital are related to nurses' opinions about nontraditional routes to parenthood, then Bao's approach makes some sense, although stratification could have been used to address this problem. One of the difficulties with this sampling plan is that we cannot be sure that Bao did not inadvertently handpick hospitals with other characteristics that might affect or be related to nurses' attitudes.

The second stage of the sampling plan involved a probability component. Within each hospital, the nursing directors were asked to select a simple random sample of 30 RNs and to distribute questionnaires to this group. Such a procedure presumably guaranteed that systematic biases would be minimized. Still, Bao cannot be sure that biases were not introduced because she herself did not control the random selection. By allowing the directors of nursing to select the sample, the investigator risked (1) the directors' misunderstanding of how to select a random sample and (2) the directors' failing to comply with the request for random selection for some reason, such as practicality or personal considerations. For example, the director might decide to exclude Ms. Pehl from the sample because of a recent death in her family. By allowing others to perform the random selection, Bao did not exercise as much control over the research situation as she might have. Furthermore, she risked additional bias stemming from low response rates in some hospitals (as low as 53% in one hospital). A personal delivery of the questionnaires and good follow-up procedures might have yielded a higher rate of returned questionnaires. Whenever response rates are low, there always remains the possibility of distortions because nonrespondents are rarely a random subsample of all possible subjects. For example, nonrespondents may be people with strong views on the issues in the questionnaire.

The key question that needs to be asked in evaluating a sampling design in a quantitative study is the following: Is the sample sufficiently representative of the population that the results can be generalized to that population? In Bao's case, it would be unwise to conclude that the opinions of the 238 nurses surveyed could be generalized to all RNs in the United States, or even to all RNs in Massachusetts. Given Bao's sampling plan, many nurses would never have had an opportunity to express their opinions. For example, unemployed nurses and RNs working in schools, community health centers, colleges, or businesses were not sampled, and their opinions might differ systematically from those working in Massachusetts hospitals. Furthermore, two hospitals refused to participate in the study, and in those that did cooperate, response rates were not high, yielding a relatively small sample size for a survey of this type.

Despite the fact that Bao's sampling plan has some limitations, it is not without merit. She did well not to rely on a single hospital from which to collect data. Furthermore, gross distortions were undoubtedly avoided by requesting nursing directors to select a random sample of nurses rather than by simply handing out questionnaires to the first 30 nurses available. Bao's results would have been enhanced had she exercised more control over sample selection and response rates, but they are nevertheless worthy of consideration. Part of the problem with the design is Bao's definition of the population. If Bao had specified a more modest target population (e.g., RNs currently employed in hospital settings in the Northeast), then her sampling plan would have had more credibility.

2. Here is a brief summary of the sampling plan of a fictitious quantitative study. Read the summary and then respond to the questions that follow.

Dolan (2001) studied the job-search strategies of recent nursing school graduates. Her survey focused on such issues as timing of job applications, number of applications, source of information about jobs, method of initial contact, and so on. She was interested in learning whether certain strategies were more successful in achieving job offers (and acceptable job offers) than others. She obtained lists of graduates from six schools of nursing in Greater Boston (two schools for each of three different types of programs). She then conducted telephone interviews with 100 graduates from each of the three program types (bachelors, diploma, and associates). Her method was to find, using local telephone directories, the telephone numbers for as many of the names on her lists as she could and to make calls until she had completed 100 interviews with graduates from each group. Thus, her final sample consisted of 300 recently graduated RNs.

Review and critique this research effort. Suggest alternative sampling designs. To assist you in your critique, here are some guiding questions:

a. What type of sampling design was used? Was this design appropriate? Would you recommend a different sampling approach? Why or why not? What are the advantages of the approach used? What are the disadvantages?

b. Identify what you believe to be the target and accessible populations in this study. How representative do you feel the accessible population is of the target population? How representative is the sample of this accessible population? What are some of the possible sources of sampling bias?

c. Did the researcher use a proportionate or disproportionate sampling plan? Is this appropriate? Why or why not?

d. Comment on the size of the sample. Does this sample size appear to be adequate?

3. Below are several suggested research articles. Read the introductory and methods sections of one or more of these articles and respond to questions a through d of Question D.2 in terms of these actual research studies.

■ Christopher, K. A. (2000). Determinants of psychological well-being in Irish immigrants. *Western Journal of Nursing Research, 22,* 123–143.

■ DeFloor, T., & Grypdonck, M. H. F. (2000). Do pressure relief cushions really relieve pressure? *Western Journal of Nursing Research, 22,* 335–350.

■ Heilemann, M.V., Lee, K. A., Stinson, J., Koshar, J. H., & Goss, G. (2000). Acculturation and perinatal health outcomes among rural women of Mexican descent. *Research in Nursing & Health, 23,* 118–125.

■ Hughes, K.K., & Dvorak, E.M. (1997). Ethical decision making. *Heart & Lung, 26,* 238–248.

■ Manogin, T. W., Bechtel, G. A., & Rami, J. S. (2000). Caring behaviors by nurses: Women's perceptions during childbirth. *Journal of Obstetric, Gynecologic, and Neonatal Nursing, 29,* 153–157.

■ Selleck, C.S., & Redding, B.A. (1998). Knowledge and attitudes of registered nurses toward perinatal substance abuse. *Journal of Obstetric, Gynecologic, and Neaonatal Nursing, 27,* 70–77.

4. A second brief summary of the sampling strategy of a fictitious study follows. Read the summary and then respond to the questions that follow.

Lombardo (2000) conducted an in-depth study of the emotional well-being of couples with fertility impairments. She conducted in-depth interviews with ten couples who were undergoing infertility treatment in a private clinic, and compared them with ten couples who had undergone such treatment and were expecting a baby. The interviews with the second group occurred in the fifth month of the pregnancies. In each of the two groups, the researcher began by selecting couples known to have had a range of experience with their fertility treatments (in terms of length and type of treatment and nature of the fertility impairment). Then, after the initial interviews were completed, the researcher recruited additional couples to saturate the theoretical lines that were developing within the data.

Review and critique this research effort. Suggest alternative sampling designs. To assist you in your critique, respond to the questions below.

a. What type of sampling strategy was used?
b. Was this sampling strategy appropriate? Would you recommend a different sampling approach? Why or why not?
c. Comment on the size of the sample. Does this sample size appear to be adequate?

5. Below are several suggested research articles. Read the introductory and methods sections of one or more of these articles and respond to parts **a** through **c** of Question D.4 in terms of these actual research studies.

- Benzein, E. G., Saveman, B., & Norberg, A. (2000). The meaning of hope in healthy, nonreligious Swedes. *Western Journal of Nursing Research, 22*, 303–319.

- Berman, R.L.H., & Iris, M.A. (1998). Approaches to self-care in late life. *Qualitative Health Research, 8*, 224–236.

- Bottorff, J. L., Johnson, J. L., Irwin, L. G., & Ratner, P. A. (2000). Narratives of smoking relapse: The stories of postpartum women. *Research in Nursing & Health, 23*, 126–134.

- Carr, J.M., & Clarke, P. (1997). Development of the concept of family vigilance. *Western Journal of Nursing Research, 19*, 726–739.

- King, G., Stewart, D., King, S., & Law, M. (2000). Organizational characteristics and issues affecting longevity of self-help groups for parents of children with special needs. *Qualitative Health Research, 10*, 225–241.

■ E. Special Projects

1. Suppose that you were interested in studying risky behavior among high school students. Describe how you might select a sample for your study using the following:

   a. A convenience sample

   b. A quota sample

   c. A cluster sample

2. Suppose you were interested in doing an in-depth study of the process of decision making regarding condom use among single men and women. Describe how you might select a sample for your study using the following:

   a. Maximum variation sample

   b. Homogeneous sample

   c. An extreme case sample

PART IV

Collection of Research Data

CHAPTER 11

Scrutinizing Data Collection Methods

■ A. Matching Exercises

1. Match each descriptive statement regarding self-report methods from Set B with one of the statements from Set A. Indicate the letter corresponding to your response next to each item in Set B.

SET A

a. An interview

b. A questionnaire

c. Both an interview and a questionnaire

d. Neither an interview nor a questionnaire

SET B   **RESPONSES**

1. Can provide respondents the protection of anonymity.   _____

2. Can be used with illiterate respondents.   _____

3. Can contain both open- and closed-ended questions.   _____

4. Is used in survey research.   _____

5. Is the best way to measure human behavior.   _____

6. Generally yields high response rates.   _____

7. Can control the order in which questions are asked
   and answered.   _____

8. Is generally an inexpensive method of data collection.   _____

9. Requires that the purpose of the study be unknown to the
   study participant.   _____

10. Is more likely to be used in qualitative studies.   _____

2. Match each problem statement from Set B with one of the statements from Set A. Indicate the letter corresponding to your response next to each item in Set B.

SET A

a. The study would *require* observational data.

b. The study *could* use observational data as well as other forms of data.

c. The study is not amenable to observational data collection.

SET B	**RESPONSES**
1. Are nurses' attitudes toward abortion related to their years of nursing experience?	_____
2. Are patients' levels of stress related to their willingness to disclose their own fears to nursing staff?	_____
3. Are the sleep-wake patterns of infants related to their gestational age at birth?	_____
4. Is the degree of physical activity of a psychiatric patient related to his or her length of hospitalization?	_____
5. Are nurses' scores on a spiritual well-being scale related to their degree of comfort in instituting spiritual nursing interventions?	_____
6. Is a child's fear during immunization related to the nurse's method of preparing the child for the shot?	_____
7. Does the presence of the father in the delivery room affect the mother's level of pain?	_____
8. Is the ability of dialysis patients to cleanse and dress their shunts related to their self-esteem and locus of control?	_____
9. Is the level of achievement motivation among nursing students related to their clinical speciality?	_____
10. Is aggressive behavior among hospitalized mentally retarded children related to styles of discipline by hospital staff?	_____

3. Match each descriptive statement regarding data collection methods from Set B with one (or more) of the statements from Set A. Indicate the letter(s) corresponding to your response next to each item in Set B.

SET A

a. Self-reports

b. Observations

c. Biophysiologic measures

d. None of the above

SET B **RESPONSES**

1. Cannot easily be gathered unobtrusively (although research purpose could be disguised). _____

2. Can be biased by the subject's desire to "look good." _____

3. Can be used to gather data from infants. _____

4. Is rarely used in qualitative studies. _____

5. Is a good way to obtain information about human *behavior*. _____

6. Data can be biased by the researcher's values and beliefs. _____

7. Can be combined with other data collection methods in a single study. _____

8. Can range from highly unstructured to highly structured data. _____

9. Can yield quantitative information. _____

10. Is the most widely used data collection method in nursing studies. _____

■ B. Completion Exercises

Write the words or phrases that correctly complete the sentences below.

1. The four dimensions along which data collection methods can vary are _____, _____, _____, and _____ .

2. _____ is the systematic gathering and critical evaluation of data relating to past occurrences.

3. When data from a previous study are reanalyzed in a new study, this is referred to as a(n) _____.

4. In a focused interview, general question areas are normally prepared in the form of a(n) _____.

5. When a group of respondents is assembled in one place to discuss questions simultaneously, the approach being used is referred to as a(n) _____.

6. _____ are narrative self-disclosures about the chronology of life experience relating to a specific topic.

7. A disadvantage of _____ questions is that the researcher may inadvertently omit some potentially important alternatives.

8. _____ questions are relatively inefficient in terms of the respondents' time.

9. If respondents are not very verbal or articulate, _____ questions are generally most appropriate.

10. A _____ is a device designed to assign scores to subjects to discriminate among them with respect to an attribute of interest.

11. Likert scales consist of a number of statements written in the _____ form.

12. In Likert scales, positively worded statements are scored in one direction, and the scoring of negatively worded statements is _____ .

13. With a semantic differential, subjects are asked to rate concepts on a series of _____ .

14. Nonresponse in self-report studies is generally not _____ and can therefore lead to bias.

15. The bias introduced when respondents select options at either end of the response continuum is known as _____ .

16. In Q sorts, forcing subjects to place a predetermined number of cards in each pile helps eliminate _____ .

17. _____ are brief narrative descriptions of people or situations to which subjects are asked to react.

18. The major focus of observation in nursing research is on human _____ .

19. The problem of behavioral distortions arising when subjects are aware that they are being observed is known as _____ .

20. The technique known as _____ involves the collection of unstructured observational data while the researcher participates in the activities of the group being observed.

21. The three major types of observational positioning in participant observation studies are _____, _____, and _____ positioning.

22. Data from unstructured observations are generally recorded on _____ and _____ .

23. In a structured observational setting, the most common procedure is to construct a(n) _____ for observed behaviors.

24. Biophysiologic measures that are taken directly within a living organism are _____ measures.

25. When physiologic materials are extracted from subjects and subjected to analysis, the data are referred to as _____ measures.

■ C. Study Questions

1. Define the following terms. Compare your definition with the definition in Chapter 11 of the textbook or in the glossary.

   a. Data collection plan _____

   _____

   b. Records _____

   _____

   c. Self-report _____

   _____

   d. Unstructured interview _____

   _____

   e. Focused interview _____

   _____

   f. Interview schedule _____

   _____

   g. Questionnaire _____

   _____

   h. Open-ended question _____

   _____

   i. Fixed-alternative question _____

   _____

   j. Visual analogue scale _____

   _____

k. Social psychological scale _____

_____

l. Response rate _____

_____

m. Response set _____

_____

n. Q sort _____

_____

o. Projective techniques _____

_____

p. Reactivity _____

_____

q. Field notes _____

_____

r. Checklist _____

_____

s. Time sampling _____

_____

t. Event sampling _____

_____

u. Biophysiologic measure _____

_____

2. Below are several research problems. Indicate what methods of data collection (self-report, observation, biophysiologic measures) you might recommend using for each. Defend your response.

a. How does an elderly patient manage the transition from hospital to

home? _____

_____

b. What are the predictors of intravenous site symptoms?_____

_____

c. What are the factors associated with smoking during pregnancy?_____

_____

d. To what extent and in what manner do nurses interact differently with male and female patients? _____

_____

e. What are the coping mechanisms of parents whose infants are long-term patients in neonatal intensive care units? _____

_____

3. Below are several research problems. Indicate which type of unstructured self-report approach you might recommend using for each. Defend your response.

a. By what process do parents of a handicapped child learn to cope with their child's problem? _____

_____

b. What are the barriers to preventive health care practices among the urban poor? _____

_____

c. What stresses does the spouse of a terminally ill patient experience?

_____

_____

d. What type of information does a nurse draw on most heavily in formulating nursing diagnoses? _____

_____

e. What are the coping mechanisms and perceived barriers to coping among severely disfigured burn patients? _____

_____

4. Below are hypothetical responses for Respondent Y and Respondent Z to the Likert statements presented in Table 11-2 of the textbook. What would the total score for both of these respondents be, using the scoring rules described in Chapter 11?

Item No.	Respondent Y	Respondent Z
1	D	SA
2	A	D
3	SA	D
4	?	A
5	D	SA
6	SA	D
Total score:	____	____

5. Below are hypothetical responses for Respondents A, B, C, and D to the Likert statements presented in Table 11-2 of the text. Three of these four sets of responses contain some indication of a possible response-set bias. Identify *which* three, and identify the types of bias.

Item No.	Respondent A	Respondent B	Respondent C	Respondent D
1	A	SA	SD	D
2	A	SD	SA	SD
3	SA	D	SA	D
4	A	A	SD	SD
5	SA	A	SD	SD
6	SA	SD	SA	D
Bias:				

6. Identify five constructs of clinical relevance that would be appropriate for measurement using a visual analogue scale (VAS).

_____

_____

_____

_____

_____

7. Below are ten research questions in which the dependent variable of interest is amenable to observation. Specify whether you think a structured or unstructured approach would be preferable and justify your response. Also, consider the extent to which reactivity might be a problem during the collection of observational data and make a recommendation regarding the degree to which the researcher should be concealed.

a. What is the effect of touch on the crying behavior of hospitalized children? _____

_____

_____

b. What is the effect of increased patient/staff ratios in psychiatric hospitals on interpersonal conflict among staff members? _____

_____

_____

c. Is the management of appetite loss in burn patients affected by nutritional information provided by nurses? _____

_____

_____

d. Is the amount and type of information transmitted at the change-of-shift report affected by the number of years of experience of the nurses? _____

_____

_____

e. Does a patient's need for personal space vary as a function of age?

_____

_____

_____

f. Are the self-grooming activities of nursing home patients related to the frequency of visits from friends and relatives? _____

_____

_____

g. Is the adequacy of a nursing student's handwashing related to his or her type of educational preparation? _____

_____

_____

h. What is the process by which very low-birth-weight infants develop the sucking response? _____

_____

_____

i. What type of patient behaviors are most likely to elicit empathic behaviors in nurses? _____

_____

_____

j. Do nurses reinforce passive behaviors among female patients more than among male patients? _____

_____

_____

8. Three nurse researchers were collaborating on a study of the effect of visits to surgical patients preoperatively by operating room nurses on the stress levels of those patients just before surgery. One researcher wanted to use the patients' self-reports on a standardized scale to measure stress; the second suggested using pulse rate; the third recommended the patients' white blood cell count. Which measure do you think would be the most appropriate for this research problem? Justify your response.

_____

_____

_____

_____

_____

■ D. Application Exercises

1. Below is a brief description of a fictitious study, followed by a critique. Do you agree with the critique? Can you add other comments relevant to

issues discussed in Chapter 11 of the textbook? (Box 11-3 offers some guiding questions.)

Fictitious Study. Pardon (2001) studied hospitalized patients' requests for nursing assistance in relation to their age, gender, and number of daily outside visitors. Her central hypothesis was that patient requests were higher among those with few or no visitors. Subjects for the study were 100 patients on a medical-surgical unit of a 500-bed hospital in New Hampshire. All 100 subjects were patients admitted for relatively routine procedures, such as appendectomies; none was terminally ill. Observations were made by the nursing staff, who were instructed to record verbatim all requests that the subjects made during a 24-hour period and all instances of patients' use of the call button. At the end of each shift, each nurse rated the patient on several dimensions, such as talkative/not talkative, hostile/friendly, and in no pain/in great pain.

Each request was then categorized according to a system that Pardon had developed. The categories included the following: request for medication; request for food or beverage; request for environmental change (e.g., temperature or light adjustment); request to see a physician; request for reading material, television, or radio; request for assistance (e.g., getting in/out of bed); and request for dialogue or emotional support. Pardon performed all of the categorizations herself based on the nurses' verbatim accounts. Pardon found that the number of patients' requests was unrelated to their gender and age, although there were age and gender differences in the types of request made. Patients with no visitors made significantly more requests than patients with one or more visitors on the day of the observation, and patients with no visitors were also somewhat more likely to be rated as unfriendly.

Critique. Pardon's decision to use an observational approach seems appropriate. Self-reports (i.e., asking patients about the frequency and type of requests they had made) would have been subject to distortions arising from memory lapse and misreporting. Patients might also have idiosyncratic notions about what constitutes a request.

Pardon elected to use a highly structured observational scheme. This decision appears to have some merit: The investigator was interested in fairly specific phenomena that lent themselves to enumeration. It is also possible, however, that a more qualitative approach would have yielded additional insights regarding why patient requests were higher among those with no visitors.

The use of both a category system and rating scales also seems to have been a good choice for capturing some information about the quantity and quality of patients' requests. The brief summary, however, does not provide a sufficient basis for evaluating whether the category system and dimensions for rating patients were appropriate. It would be useful to know how they were developed. Here again, a series of unstructured observations might have provided a rich basis for the development of relevant behavioral codes and dimensions of patient characteristics.

Several other aspects of Pardon's study could have been improved. First, consider the possibility of reactivity. It is likely that patients were not informed about their participation while the data were being collected, which in this case seems appropriate; the privacy of the patients was not seriously threatened, and patients would undoubtedly have altered their interactions with the nursing staff if they had known that their dialogue was being scrutinized. Thus, Pardon's procedure of having nurses record patients' requests after they were made (i.e., after leaving the patients' rooms) eliminated the problem of reactivity stemming from the patient. But what about the reactivity of the nurses? The nurses knew exactly what the researcher was studying and could have communicated cues to the patients in subtle or not-so-subtle ways. The nurses' nonverbal behavior could have either encouraged or discouraged patients' requests for assistance.

Two other problems relate to the use of the nurses as the observational recorders. First, unless the nurses were thoroughly trained, some might have misinterpreted the researcher's definition of requests. Second, the nurses were required to report verbatim the patients' requests, an activity that is by no means easy, particularly for those whose main priority is patient care. In many cases, the nurses probably did not remember accurately the wording of the patients' questions.

From a methodologic point of view, the best procedure would have been to tape-record all nurse–patient dialogue unobtrusively. In addition to providing accuracy and eliminating the risk of nurse reactivity, the use of a recording device would have permitted more fine-grained analyses of the content and tone of the requests. However, concealed recording equipment would be ethically problematic. Perhaps the researcher could have told both the nursing staff and subjects about the presence of recording equipment and described only in broad terms the nature of the study (e.g., to understand patient–nurse communication patterns better).

Pardon sampled an entire 24-hour period for all 100 subjects. It would probably have been wiser to sample 1-hour segments over a 48-hour to 72-hour interval. A single day may not have adequately represented the range of patient requests during a hospital stay and could also have been atypical in terms of visitation.

Pardon elected to categorize patient communication that took the form of requests for assistance. This system covered all types of request, but no other patient conversation. Although the decision to use such a nonexhaustive category scheme is understandable, it does have the disadvantage of failing to provide a context for understanding patient behavior. If a patient made 15 requests in 1 day, it might be useful to know whether these requests represented all patient-initiated communication or only a small fraction of it.

Categorization of the requests was handled centrally by Pardon rather than by individual nurse observers. This approach has the advantage of not introducing different biases from different coders. It does mean, however, that any biases went undetected. Pardon would have been well-advised to have a second person categorize the requests (or at least a portion of them) to determine agreement among different coders.

With respect to this latter issue, the use of nurses from all three shifts who rated patients' communication or to record actual dialogue would have provided yet another opportunity to verify nurses' observations independently. In summary, then, Pardon's data collection plan was fairly well conceived but could also have been improved in a number of respects, including the judicious use of unstructured observations and possibly unstructured self-reports (e.g., interviews with patients who made many or few requests) to facilitate interpretation of the results.

2. Here is a brief summary of a fictitious study. Read the summary and then respond to the questions that follow.

Leidig (2001) conducted a survey that focused on drug use patterns in an urban adolescent population. The survey used self-administered questionnaires that were distributed to 25 high schools and administered in group (home-room) sessions to 3568 respondents. The questionnaire consisted of 56 closed-ended and 2 open-ended questions. Included were background questions; questions on the students' attitudes toward, knowledge of, and experience with various drugs; and questions on the students' physical and mental health. The instrument was pretested with 10 community college students before final administration of the survey.

Review and critique the above description of the overall study. Suggest possible alternative ways of collecting the data for the research problem. To assist you in your critique, here are some guiding questions. (Review also the critiquing guidelines in Box 11-1 of the textbook.)

a. The data in this study were collected by self-report. Could the data have been collected in another way? *Should* they have been, in your opinion?

b. Were the data collected by questionnaire or interview? Was the decision to use this method appropriate, or would you recommend an alternative procedure? Comment on the advantages and disadvantages of the procedure used for this particular research problem.

c. Comment on the degree of structure of the instrument used. Would you recommend a more structured or a less structured instrument? Why or why not?

d. Was the instrument adequately pretested?

e. Comment on the method in which the instrument was administered. Was the method efficient? Did it yield an adequate response rate? Did it appear costly?

3. Below are several suggested research articles. Skim one or more of these articles, paying particular attention to the methods used to collect the self-report data. Then respond to questions a through e from Question D.2 in terms of this actual research study.

■ Mahon, N. E., Yarcheski, A., & Yarcheski, T. J. (2000). Positive and negative outcomes of anger in early adolescents. *Research in Nursing & Health, 23,* 17–24.

■ O'Farrell, P., Murray, J., & Hotz, S. B. (2000). Psychologic distress among spouses of patients undergoing cardiac rehabilitation. *Heart & Lung, 29,* 97–104.

■ Stordeur, S., Vandenberghe, C., & D'hoore, W. (2000). Leadership styles across hierarchical levels in nursing departments. *Nursing Research, 49,* 37–43.

4. Another brief summary of a fictitious study is presented next. Read the summary and then respond to the questions that follow.

Sacks and Carter (2000) undertook an in-depth study of parents' experiences caring for children dying of cancer. The project was designed to describe the evolution of parents' caring practices in response to the demands of living with a dying child. The researchers conducted totally unstructured interviews with each parent separately, beginning with the grand tour question, "Tell me about what happened when you first learned that your child was ill." Subsequently, Sacks and Carter conducted a more focused interview with both parents together (in homes where there were two parents). All interviews were tape recorded and later transcribed for analysis. The researchers also spent 30 hours in each home in 10 separate sessions over a two-month period observing parental caring practices. Most of the observations occurred in the child's bedroom or in a family/living room. The observations focused on the following aspects of a caregiving episode: the context for the episode, the nature and content of any interactions, the activities that occurred; how the activities unfolded; and what the outcomes of the activities were. All observational notes were written out in full shortly after the observational sessions and the notes were later transcribed.

Review and critique this study. Suggest alternative ways of collecting the data for the research problem. To assist you in your critique, here are some guiding questions. (Refer also to the questions in Boxes 11-1 and 11-2 of the textbook.)

   a. The data in this study were collected through in-depth interviews and observation. Could the data have been collected in another way? *Should* they have been, in your opinion?
   b. Was the amount of structure in the data collection appropriate, or should there have been more or less structure?
   c. Comment on the method in which the data were collected (e.g., the setting, the use of tape recorders, etc.)
   d. What types of biases do you think might be operational in this study?

5. Below are several suggested research articles. Skim one or more of these articles, paying particular attention to the methods used to collect the data. Then respond to questions a through d from Question D.4 in terms of this actual research study.

   ■ Dougherty, C. M., Benoliel, J. Q., & Bellin, C. (2000). Domains of nursing intervention after sudden cardiac arrest and automatic internal cardioverter defibrillator implantation. *Heart & Lung, 29,* 79–86.

- Foley, B. J., Minick, P., & Kee, C. (2000). Nursing advocacy during a military operation. *Western Journal of Nursing Research, 22*, 492–507.
- McSweeney, J. C., & Crane, P. B. (2000). Challenging the rules: Women's prodomal and acute symptoms of myocardial infarction. *Research in Nursing & Health, 23*, 135–146.
- Rosenfeld, A., & Gilkeson, J. (2000). Meaning of illness for women with coronary heart disease. *Heart & Lung, 29*, 105–112.
- Whittemore, R., Rankin, S. H., Callahan, C. D., Leder, M. C., & Carroll, D. L. (2000). The peer advisor experience providing social support. *Qualitative Health Research, 10*, 260–276.

6. A brief summary of a fictitious observational study follows. Read the summary and then respond to the questions that follow.

Meany (2000) studied the effect of a school nutritional program on the snacking behaviors of students in grades 1 through 6. During the month of October, the experimental program (which consisted of discussion groups led by the school nurse, posters, and classroom activities initiated by the teachers) was introduced into two elementary schools in a large Eastern city. Two other schools were used as the controls. The children in all four schools were observed with respect to their selection of snack foods, offered once a week at a 2:00 pm snack break. Each snack selected was rated in terms of its nutritional value on a scale from 1 to 9. The observations were made by the school nurses who were in the classrooms and noted the selection of each student. Observations were made during the months of October (when the program was implemented) and November (after the program was completed). The data consisted of two main types of information: (1) the frequency with which each snack item was selected each week; and (2) the nutritional ratings for the selected snacks for each child. An analysis of these data revealed that the children in the experimental classrooms selected significantly fewer snacks categorized as "nonnutritional salty snacks" (e.g., potato chips) and had a significantly higher average nutritional rating in November than children in the comparison classrooms.

Review and critique this study. Suggest alternative ways of collecting the data for the research problem. To assist you in your critique, here are some guiding questions:

a. The data in this study were collected by observation. Could the data have been collected in another way? *Should* they have been, in your opinion?

b. Specify the relationship between the observer and those being observed with regard to concealment. Do you feel that the specified relationship was appropriate?

c. Would you classify the study as having used an unstructured or structured observational procedure? Was the amount of structure in the data collection appropriate, or should there have been more or less structure?

d. Was the specific procedure used to capture the study variables an adequate way to operationalize the variables? Could you recommend any improvements?

e. What type of sampling plan was used to sample observations in this study? Would an alternative sampling plan have been better? Why or why not?

f. What types of observational bias do you think might be operational in this study?

g. Comment on the appropriateness of the individuals who made the observations. Can you identify any potential problems with respect to the internal and external validity of the study?

7. Below are several suggested research articles in which an observational approach was used. Review one of the articles and respond to questions **a** through **g** from Question D.6, to the extent possible, in terms of this study.

■ Dickson, G. (2000). Aboriginal grandmothers' experience with health promotion and participatory action research. *Qualitative Health Research, 10,* 188–213.

■ Emami, A., Torres, S., Lipson, J. G., & Ekman, S. (2000). An ethnographic study of a day care center for Iranian immigrant seniors. *Western Journal of Nursing Research, 22,* 169–188.

■ Holditch-Davis, D., Miles, M. S., & Belyea, M. (2000). Feeding and nonfeeding interactions of mothers and prematures. *Western Journal of Nursing Research, 22,* 320–334.

■ Rateau, M. R. (2000). Confusion and aggression in restrained elderly persons undergoing hip repair surgery. *Applied Nursing Research, 13,* 50–54.

■ Thomas, K. A. (2000). Differential effects of breast- and formula-feeding on preterm infants' sleep-wake patterns. *Journal of Obstetric, Gynecologic, and Neonatal Nursing, 29,* 145–152.

8. A summary of another fictitious study follows next. Read the summary and then respond to the questions that follow.

Lebowitz (2000) conducted a quasi-experimental study of the effectiveness of a program for treating the physiologic anemia associated with pregnancy. The experimental treatment involved instruction regarding a nutritional regimen. The experimental group received verbal instructions by a nurse-midwife regarding dietary requirements and a list of foods known to be high in iron. Recommended daily amounts of certain foods were prescribed. The intervention also involved follow-up telephone conversations with the experimental group members at the 30th and 34th weeks of the pregnancy to discuss dietary and nutritional concerns. The comparison group members were given information that is normally given to pregnant women, with no individual follow-up. Fifty pregnant women who were outpatients at one hospital clinic served as the experimental subjects, and 50 pregnant women who were clients at a health maintenance organization served as the comparison group subjects. Lebowitz chose hematocrit readings as the measure of effectiveness of the experimental intervention. During the sixth month of the pregnancy, and again at the 36th-week visit, a hematocrit laboratory test was performed. The data were analyzed by comparing the degree of change that had occurred in the two hematocrit readings within the two groups. The researcher found no significant differences in physiologic anemia in the two groups, as measured by the changes in hematocrit tests.

Review and critique this study. Suggest alternative ways of collecting the data for the research problem. To assist you in your critique, here are some guiding questions:

a. The data in this study were collected by a biophysiologic measure. Could the data have been collected in another way? In your opinion, should they have been?
b. Is the measure used an in vivo or in vitro type of measurement? Is it an invasive or noninvasive type of procedure?
c. Comment on the objectivity of the data collection method. How does its objectivity compare with other methods of measuring the dependent variable (e.g., observations of pallor of the skin, mucous membranes, and fingernail beds)?
d. What other biophysiologic measures might have been used to collect data in the study?

9. Below are several suggested research articles in which a biophysiologic method was used. Review one of the articles, and respond to questions **a** through **d** from Question D.8, to the extent possible, in terms of this actual study.

   ■ Christman, S. K., Fish, A. F., Bernhard, L., Frid, D. J., Smith, B. A., & Mitchell, G. L. (2000). Continuous handrail support, oxygen uptake, and heart rate in women during submaximal step treadmill exercise. *Research in Nursing & Health, 23,* 35–42.

   ■ Fontana, J. A. (2000). The energy costs of a modified form of T'ai Chi exercise. *Nursing Research, 49,* 91–96.

   ■ Kang, D. H., Coe, C. L., Karaszewski, J., & McCarthy, D. O. (1998). Relationship of social support to stress responses and immune function in healthy and asthmatic adolescents. *Research in Nursing & Health, 21,* 117–128.

   ■ Larson, E., et al. (2000). Assessment of alternative hand hygiene regimens to improve skin health among neonatal intensive care unit nurses. *Heart & Lung, 29,* 136–142.

   ■ McCarthy, D. O. et al. (1998). Mereperidine attenuates the secretion but not the transcription of interleuken 1β in human mononuclear leukocytes. *Nursing Research, 47,* 19–24.

■ E. Special Projects

1. Develop a topic guide for studying barriers to health-care utilization among the urban poor.

2. Suggest one open-ended and one closed-ended question relating to each of the following variables. Compare the quality and amount of information that could be obtained with each.

   a. Women's attitudes toward nurse-midwives

   b. Factors influencing a decision to obtain a vasectomy

   c. Perceived adequacy of community health care services

   d. Student nurses' first experiences with the death of a patient

   e. Factors influencing nurses' administration of pain-relieving narcotics to patients

3. Develop a research question for an observational study. Make a recommendation regarding the use of a structured or unstructured approach for this problem.

_____

_____

_____

_____

_____

4. Suppose that you wanted to evaluate the effect of an experimental nursing intervention on the well-being and comfort of cardiac patients. Indicate several physiologic measures you might consider using in such a study. Evaluate each of your suggestions with respect to ease of obtaining the data, relevance, and objectivity.

_____

_____

_____

_____

_____

5. Using procedures described in Chapter 11, suggest methods of collecting data on the following: fear of death among the elderly; body image among amputees; reactions to the onset of menarche; nurses' morale in an emergency room; and dependence among children with cerebral palsy.

_____

_____

_____

_____

_____

CHAPTER 12

Evaluating Measurements and Data Quality

■ A. Matching Exercises

1. Match each statement from Set B with one of the phrases from Set A. Indicate the letter corresponding to your response next to each of the statements in Set B.

SET A

a. Reliability

b. Validity

c. Both reliability and validity

d. Neither reliability nor validity

SET B   **RESPONSES**

1. Is concerned with the accuracy of measures.   _____

2. The measures must be high on this for the results of a study to be valid.   _____

3. If a measure possesses this, then it is necessarily valid.   _____

4. Can in some cases be estimated by procedures that yield a quantified coefficient.   _____

5. Can be enhanced by lengthening (adding subparts to) the scale.   _____

6. May in some cases be assessed by scrutinizing the components (subparts) of the measure.   _____

7. Is necessarily high when the measure is high on objectivity.   _____

8. Is concerned with whether the researcher has adequately conceptualized the variables under investigation.   _____

2. Match each statement from Set B with one of the phrases from Set A. Indicate the letter corresponding to your response next to each of the statements in Set B.

SET A

a. Data triangulation

b. Investigator triangulation

c. Theory triangulation

d. Method triangulation

SET B   **RESPONSES**

1. A researcher studying health beliefs of the rural elderly interviews old people and health care providers in the area.   _____

2. A researcher tests narrative data, collected in interviews with people who attempted suicide, against two alternative explanations of stress and coping.   _____

3. Two researchers independently interview 10 informants in a study of adjustment to a cancer diagnosis and debrief with each other to review what they have learned.   _____

4. A researcher studying school-based clinics observes interactions in the clinics and also conducts in-depth interviews with students.   _____

5. A researcher studying the process of resolving an infertility problem interviews husbands and wives separately.   _____

6. Themes emerging in the field notes of an observer on a psychiatric ward are categorized and labeled independently by the researcher and an assistant.   _____

■ B. Completion Exercises

Write the words or phrases that correctly complete the sentences below.

1. People are not measured directly; their _____ are measured.

2. The procedure known as _____ refers to the assignment of numerical information to communicate how much of an attribute is present.

3. In measurement, numbers are assigned according to specified _____
_____.

4. From a measurement perspective, response-set biases represent a source
of _____.

5. A reliable measure is one that maximizes the _____
component of observed scores.

6. Test-retest reliability focuses on the _____
of a measure.

7. The most widely used index of internal consistency reliability is _____
_____.

8. Procedures that examine the proportion of agreements between two independent judges yield estimates of _____.

9. An instrument that is not reliable cannot be _____.

10. A measure that looks as though it is measuring what it purports to measure is said to have _____ validity.

11. The type of validity that focuses on the representativeness of the subparts of a measure is _____ validity.

12. The type of validity that deals with the ability of an instrument to distin-
guish individuals who differ in terms of some future criterion is _____
_____ validity.

13. The known-groups technique is a method used to evaluate an instrument's _____ validity.

14. A(n) _____ is a process under-
taken specifically to assess the reliability and validity of an instrument.

15. The four criteria for establishing the trustworthiness of qualitative data
are _____, _____,
_____, and _____ .

16. When a qualitative researcher undertakes a(n) _____
in the field, he or she has more opportunity to develop trust with informants and to test for possible misinformation.

17. The use of multiple sources of information in a study as a means of verification is known as _____.

18. The technique of debriefing with informants to evaluate the credibility of
qualitative data is referred to as a(n) _____.

19. The criterion of _____ refers to the
objectivity or neutrality of the data.

20. In qualitative studies, a(n)_____ by an independent reviewer can verify the dependability and neutrality of the data and their interpretation.

■ C. Study Questions

1. Define the following terms. Compare your definition with the definition in Chapter 12 of the textbook or in the glossary.

   a. Measurement _____

   _____

   b. Obtained score _____

   _____

   c. Error of measurement _____

   _____

   d. Reliability _____

   _____

   e. Test-retest reliability _____

   _____

   f. Reliability coefficient _____

   _____

   g. Internal consistency _____

   _____

   h. Cronbach's alpha _____

   _____

   i. Interrater reliability _____

   _____

   j. Validity _____

   _____

   k. Content validity _____

   _____

   l. Criterion-related validity _____

   _____

m. Construct validity _____

_____

n. Known-groups technique _____

_____

o. Triangulation _____

_____

p. Audit trail _____

_____

q. Credibility _____

_____

r. Persistent observation _____

_____

s. Transferability _____

_____

2. The reliability of measures of which of the following attributes would *not* be appropriately assessed using a test-retest procedure with one month between administrations. Why?

a. Attitudes toward abortion _____

_____

b. Stress _____

_____

c. Achievement motivation _____

_____

d. Nursing effectiveness _____

_____

e. Depression _____

_____

3. Comment on the meaning and implications of the following statement: A researcher found that the internal consistency of her 20-item scale measuring attitudes toward nurse-midwives was .74, using the Cronbach alpha formula.

_____

_____

_____

_____

_____

4. In the following situation, what might be some of the sources of measurement error?

> One hundred nurses who worked in a large metropolitan hospital were asked to complete a 10-item Likert scale designed to measure job satisfaction. The questionnaires were distributed by nursing supervisors at the end of shifts. The staff nurses were asked to complete the forms and return them immediately to their supervisors.

_____

_____

_____

_____

_____

5. Identify what is incorrect about the following statements:

a. "My scale is highly reliable, so it must be valid." _____

_____

b. "My instrument yielded an internal consistency coefficient of .80, so it must be stable." _____

_____

c. "The validity coefficient between my scale and a criterion measure was .40; therefore, my scale must be of low validity." _____

_____

d. "The validation study proved that my measure has construct validity."

_____

_____

e. "My measure of stress was highly reliable in my study of primiparous women; you should use it in your study of stress among emergency room staff." _____

_____

■ D. Application Exercises

1. Below is a brief description of a fictitious study, followed by a critique. Do you agree with the critique? Can you add other comments relevant to issues discussed in Chapter 12 of the textbook? (Box 12-1 offers some guiding questions.)

Fictitious Study. Fox (2000) developed a scale that measured feelings of loneliness and social isolation among the elderly. She developed twelve Likert statements, six of which were worded positively and the other six of which were worded negatively. Examples include, "I have lots of friends with whom I am close" and "Sometimes days go by without my having a real conversation with anyone." Fox pretested her instrument with 50 men and women aged 60 to 70 years living independently in the community. She estimated the reliability of the scale using internal consistency procedures (Cronbach's alpha), which yielded a reliability coefficient of .61.

Fox took two steps to validate her scale. First, she asked two geriatric nurses to examine the 12 items to assess the scale's content validity. These experts suggested some wording changes on three items and recommended replacing one other. Next, she compared the scale scores of 100 elderly widows and widowers with 100 elderly married men and women. Her rationale was that the widowed would probably feel lonelier as a group than the nonwidowed. Her expectation was confirmed. Fox concluded that her scale was sufficiently valid and reliable.

Critique. Fox took some reasonable steps in constructing her scale and assessing its quality. For example, Fox's scale was counterbalanced with negative and positive statements, thereby reducing the risk of measurement error attributable to acquiescence response bias. It appears that she included a sufficient number of items (12) to yield discriminating scores. She used the Cronbach's alpha approach, which is the best method available for assessing the internal consistency of Likert scales.

The reliability of Fox's scale, however, could and should be improved. The reliability coefficient of .61 suggests that there is considerable measurement error. There are several steps that Fox could take to try to raise the reliability. First, she could make sure that each item on her scale is doing the job it was intended to do. Remember that scales are designed to discriminate among people who possess different amounts of some trait, in this case social isolation. If Fox identifies one or more items for which there is little variability (*i.e.,* most respondents either agree or disagree), then the item should be discarded. It is probably not measuring social isolation if everyone responds the same way.

Next, Fox could make sure that her scoring procedure is correct. Her assignment of scores is based on a *judgment* of what is a positively and negatively worded item. Respondents with high scores should agree with the positively worded items and disagree with the negatively worded ones. If substantial numbers of people did the opposite, either the item should be eliminated or perhaps the scoring should be reversed. If people with high scores are divided in their agreement with an item, this could be caused by ambiguity in the wording of that question, so perhaps it should be revised. Finally, Fox should consider lengthening the scale. Other things being equal, longer scales are more reliable than shorter ones.

Fox's efforts to validate her scale also deserve comment. Her first step was to consider the content validity of the scale. Having two knowledgeable people examine the scale was a very desirable thing to do. Nevertheless, it cannot be said that this activity in itself ensured the validity of the scale. As a second step, Fox used the known-groups technique. The data she obtained provided some useful evidence of the scale's construct validity. After making some of the revisions suggested above to improve the scale's reliability, however, Fox would do well to gather some additional data to support the scale's construct validity. For example, one might suspect that people would feel less socially isolated if they reported having kin living within a 20-mile radius; if they had visited with a friend within a 72-hour period preceding the completion of the scale; and if they were active members of a club, church group, or other social organization. All of these expectations could be tested. If Fox took these additional steps to establish the reliability and validity of her scale and obtained favorable results, she could be justifiably confident that the quality of her scale was high.

2. A brief summary of a fictitious study is presented next. Read the summary and then respond to the questions that follow.

Whann (2001) was interested in studying paternal bonding and attachment among men who had recently become fathers. Her main objective was to compare paternal attachment among men who had participated with their wives in prenatal classes and were present during childbirth with men who had not. In reviewing prior work in this area, Whann was unable to identify a paternal attachment scale that she found suitable to her needs. Therefore, she developed her own scale to measure paternal attachment. Her scale consisted of 10 statements that respondents were asked to rate as "very much like me," "somewhat like me," or "not at all like me." An example of the statements on the scale is, "The birth of my baby aroused sentiments of immediate affection, closeness, and pride." Total scores were obtained by using procedures analogous to those used for summated rating scales. Whann pretested her scale with 30 men within 48 hours of the delivery of their babies. The internal consistency of the scale was assessed using the split-half technique, which yielded a reliability coefficient of .62. In terms of validating the instrument, Whann used two approaches. First, she invited two colleagues who worked in maternal-child nursing to review the 10 statements and evaluate them in terms of content validity. Second, she asked nurses who worked in the hospital maternity ward to provide ratings, on a 0 to 10 scale, of how attached each new father appeared to be, based on the nurses' observations of the fathers' behavior regarding their babies. The correlations between the fathers' scale scores and the nurses' ratings was .56.

Review and critique this research effort. Suggest alternative ways of assessing the reliability and validity of the instrument. To assist you in your critique, here are some guiding questions:

a. What method was used to assess the reliability of the instrument? On what aspect of reliability does this method focus? Is this focus appropriate? Should some alternative method for estimating reliability have been used? Should an *additional* method of estimating reliability have been used?

b. Comment on the adequacy of the instrument's reliability. Should the reliability be better? If so, what might the researcher do to improve the reliability?

c. What method was used to assess the validity of the instrument? On what aspect of validity does this approach focus? Is this focus appropriate? Should some alternative method for estimating validity have been used? Should an *additional* method of estimating validity have been used?

d. Comment on the adequacy of the instrument's validity. Should the validity be better? If so, what might the researcher do to improve the validity?

3. Below are several suggested research articles. Read one of these articles, paying special attention to the ways the researcher assessed the adequacy of his or her measuring tool. Evaluate the measurement strategy, using questions a through d from Question D.2 as a guide. (Ignore the more technical aspects of the report, such as those that deal with factor analysis.)

■ Fuller, B. F., & Neu, M. (2000). Validity and reliability of a practice-based infant pain assessment instrument. *Clinical Nursing Research, 9,* 124–143.

■ Irvine, D., O'Brien-Pallas, L. L., Murray, M., Cockerill, R., Sidani, S., Laurie-Shaw, B., & Lochhaas-Gerlach, J. (2000). The reliability and validity of two health status measures for evaluating outcomes of home care nursing. *Research in Nursing & Health, 23,* 43–54.

■ Resnick, B., & Jenkins, L. S. (2000). Testing the reliability and validity of the Self-Efficacy for Exercise Scale. *Nursing Research, 49,* 154–159.

■ Ryden, M. B., Gross, C. R., Savik, K., Snyder, M., Oh, H. L., Jang, Y., Wang, J., Krichbaum, K. E. (2000). Development of a measure of resident satisfaction with the nursing home. *Research in Nursing & Health, 23,* 237–245.

4. Below are several suggested research reports on qualitative studies.

■ Draucker, C. B., & Stern, P. N. (2000). Women's responses to sexual violence by male intimates. *Western Journal of Nursing Research, 22,* 385–406.

■ Hupcey, J. E. (1998). Establishing the nurse-family relationship in the intensive care unit. *Western Journal of Nursing Research, 20,* 180–194.

- LaCharity, L. A. (1997). The experiences of postmenopausal women with coronary artery disease. *Western Journal of Nursing Research, 19,* 583–607.
- Weiss, J., & Hutchinson, S. A. (2000). Warnings about vulnerability in clients with diabetes and hypertension. *Qualitative Health Research, 10,* 521–537.

Read and critique one of these articles, paying special attention to the ways in which the researcher addressed data quality issues. To assist you in your critique, here are some guiding questions:

a. Does the report discuss efforts the researcher made to enhance and appraise data quality? Is the documentation regarding efforts to assess data quality sufficiently detailed and clear?

b. What were those efforts? Was any type of triangulation used? Were there member checks? Was there an external audit of the data?

c. How adequate were the procedures that were used? What other techniques could have been used profitably to enhance and assess data quality? How much confidence do the researcher's efforts inspire regarding data quality?

d. Given the procedures that were used to enhance data quality, what can you conclude about the credibility, transferability, dependability, and confirmability of the data?

■ E. Special Projects

1. Suppose that you were developing an instrument to measure attitudes toward human cloning. Your measure consists of 15 Likert-type items. Describe what you would do to (a) estimate the reliability of your scale and (b) assess the validity of your scale.

2. Suggest the type of groups that might be used to validate measures of the following concepts using the known-groups technique:

   a. Self-esteem

   b. Empathy

   c. Capacity for self-care

   d. Emotional dependence

   e. Depression

   f. Hopelessness

   g. Health-promoting practices

   h. Health motivation

   i. Body image

   j. Coping capacity

3. Suppose you were interested in conducting an in-depth study of coping strategies among women who had been raped. Describe ways in which you might achieve: (a) data triangulation, (b) method triangulation, (c) member checks.

PART V

Analysis of Research Data

CHAPTER 13

Analyzing Quantitative Data

■ A. Matching Exercises

1. Match each variable in Set B with the level of measurement from Set A that captures the highest possible level for that variable. Indicate the letter corresponding to your response next to each variable in Set B.

SET A

a. Nominal scale

b. Ordinal scale

c. Interval scale

d. Ratio scale

SET B   **RESPONSES**

1. Hours spent in labor before childbirth. _____

2. Religious affiliation. _____

3. Time to first postoperative voiding. _____

4. Responses to a single Likert scale item. _____

5. Temperature on the centigrade scale. _____

6. Nursing specialty area. _____

7. Status on the following scale: in poor health; in fair health; in good health; in excellent health. _____

8. Pulse rate. _____

9. Score on a 25-item Likert scale. _____

10. Highest college degree attained (bachelor's, master's, doctorate). _____

11. Apgar scores. _____

12. Membership in the American Nurses' Association. _____

2. Match each statement or phrase from Set B with one of the phrases from Set A. Indicate the letter corresponding to your response next to each of the statements in Set B.

SET A

a. Measure(s) of central tendency
b. Measure(s) of variability
c. Measure(s) of neither central tendency nor variability
d. Measure(s) of both central tendency and variability

SET B   **RESPONSES**

  1. The range.   _____

  2. In lay terms, an average.   _____

  3. A percentage.   _____

  4. Descriptor(s) of a distribution of scores.   _____

  5. Descriptor(s) of how heterogeneous a set of values is.   _____

  6. The standard deviation.   _____

  7. The mode.   _____

  8. The median.   _____

  9. A normal distribution.   _____

 10. The mean.   _____

3. Match each phrase or statement from Set B with one of the phrases in Set A. Indicate the letter corresponding to your response next to each of the statements in Set B.

SET A

a. Parametric test
b. Nonparametric test
c. Neither parametric nor nonparametric tests
d. Both parametric and nonparametric tests

SET B   **RESPONSES**

  1. The chi-squared test.   _____

  2. Paired *t*-test.   _____

  3. Researcher establishes the risk of Type I errors.   _____

SET B   **RESPONSES**

4. Used when a score distribution is markedly nonnormal.   _____

5. Offers proof that the null hypothesis is either true or false.   _____

6. Assumes the dependent variable is measured on an interval or ratio scale.   _____

7. Uses sample data to estimate population values.   _____

8. ANOVA.   _____

9. Computed statistics are compared to tabled values based on theoretical distributions.   _____

10. Pearson's *r*.   _____

■ B. Completion Exercises

Write the words or phrases that correctly complete the sentence below.

1. Nominal measurement involves a simple _____ of objects according to some criterion.

2. Rank-order questions are an example of _____ measures.

3. With ratio-level measures there is a real, rational _____.

4. Unlike ordinal measures, interval measures involve _____ _____ between points on the scale.

5. A descriptive index (e.g., percentage) from a population is called a(n) _____.

6. A(n) _____ is a systematic arrangement of quantitative data from lowest to highest values.

7. _____ are a common way of presenting frequency information in graphic form.

8. A distribution is described as _____ if the two halves are *mirror* images of each other.

9. A distribution is described as _____ skewed if its longer tail points to the left.

10. A distribution that has only one peak is said to be _____ _____.

11. Many human characteristics, such as height and intelligence, are distributed to approximate a(n) _____.

12. Measures that summarize the typical value in a distribution are known as measures of _____.

13. Measures of _____ are concerned with how spread out the data are.

14. When scores are not very spread out (*i.e.*, dispersed over a wide range of values), the sample is said to be _____ with respect to that variable.

15. The most widely used measure of variability is the _____ _____.

16. Descriptive statistics for two variables examined simultaneously are called _____.

17. Relationships are described as _____ if high values on one variable are associated with low values on a second.

18. The most commonly used correlation index is _____ _____.

19. Researchers using quantitative analysis apply _____ _____ to draw conclusions about a population based on information from a sample.

20. Sampling distributions of means have a _____ distribution.

21. The degree of risk of making a _____ error is controlled by the researcher.

22. Tests that involve the estimation of parameters are referred to as _____ _____ tests.

23. The most commonly used _____ are the .05 and .01 levels.

24. Using $\alpha = .01$ rather than $\alpha = .05$ level *increases* the risk of committing a _____ error.

25. The statistic computed in an analysis of variance is the _____ _____ statistic.

26. When both the independent and dependent variables are nominal measures, the test statistic usually calculated is the _____ _____.

27. The analysis that would be used to predict patients' postoperative fatigue levels on the basis of three preoperative characteristics would be _____ _____.

28. The square of _____ indicates the proportion of variance accounted for in a dependent variable by several independent variables.

29. Multiple correlation coefficients can range in value from _____ to _____.

30. ANCOVA is shorthand for _____.

31. In ANCOVA, the extraneous variable being controlled is referred to as the _____.

32. The multivariate procedure used to reduce a large number of variables to a smaller set of unified dimensions is _____.

33. If the independent variables were gender, age, and cigarette smoking status and the dependent variable were lung cancer status (ever had/never had), the analysis could either be _____ or _____.

34. The procedure known as _____ transforms the probability of an event occurring into an odds ratio.

35. Two procedures that are used in causal modeling are _____ and _____.

■ C. Study Questions

1. Define the following terms. Use the textbook to compare your definition with the definition in Chapter 13 or in the Glossary.

   a. Level of measurement _____

   _____

   b. Statistic _____

   _____

   c. Skewed distribution _____

   _____

   d. Bimodal distribution _____

   _____

e. Normal distribution _____

_____

f. Median _____

_____

g. Mean _____

_____

h. Standard deviation _____

_____

i. Correlation coefficient _____

_____

j. Sampling error _____

_____

k. Sampling distribution _____

_____

l. Standard error of the mean _____

_____

m. Type I error _____

_____

n. Type II error _____

_____

o. Level of significance _____

_____

p. Statistical significance _____

_____

q. Nonparametric tests _____

_____

r. *t*-test _____

_____

s. Analysis of variance _____

_____

    t. Chi-squared test _____

_____

    u. Multivariate statistics _____

_____

    v. Multiple regression analysis _____

_____

    w. Analysis of covariance _____

_____

2. Name five physiologic measures that yield ratio-level measurements.

    a. _____

    b. _____

    c. _____

    d. _____

    e. _____

3. Prepare a frequency distribution and frequency polygon for the set of
scores below, which represent the ages of 30 women receiving estrogen
replacement therapy:

    47 50 51 50 48 51 50 51 49 51
    54 49 49 53 51 52 51 52 50 53
    49 51 52 51 50 55 48 54 53 52

Describe the resulting distribution in terms of its symmetry and modality
(*i.e.*, whether it is unimodal or multimodal).

_____

_____

_____

_____

_____

4. Calculate the mean, median, and mode for the following pulse rates:

   78 84 69 98 102 72 87 75 79 84 88 84 83 71 73

   Mean _____

   Median _____

   Mode _____

5. A group of nurse researchers measured the amount of time (in minutes) spent in recreational activities by a sample of 200 hospitalized paraplegic patients. They compared male and female patients as well as those aged 50 and younger versus those over 50 years old. The four group means (50 subjects per group) were as follows:

Age	Male	Female
≤ 50 years	98.2	70.1
>50	50.8	68.3

A two-way ANOVA yielded the following results

	F	df	p
Sex	3.61	1, 196	NS
Age group	5.87	1, 196	<.05
Sex × Age group	6.96	1, 196	<.01

Interpret the meaning of these results.

_____

_____

_____

_____

_____

6. The correlation between the number of days absent per year and annual salary in a sample of 100 employees of an insurance company was found to be −.23 ($p < .05$). Discuss this result in terms of its meaning.

_____

_____

_____

_____

_____

7. Indicate which statistical tests you would use to analyze data for the following variables:

   a. Variable 1 is psychiatric patients' gender; variable 2 is whether the patient has attempted suicide in the past 6 months. _____

   _____

   b. Variable 1 is the participation versus nonparticipation of patients with a pulmonary embolus in a special treatment group; variable 2 is the pH of the patients' arterial blood gases. _____

   _____

   c. Variable 1 is serum creatinine concentration levels; variable 2 is daily urine output. _____

   _____

   d. Variable 1 is patient's marital status (married versus divorced/separated/widowed versus never married); variable 2 is the patients' degree of self-reported depression (measured on a 30-item depression scale).

   _____

   _____

8. Suggest possible covariates that could be used to control extraneous variation in the following analyses:

   a. An analysis of the effect of family income on the incidence of child abuse _____

   _____

b. An analysis of the effect of age on patients' acceptance of pastoral counseling _____

_____

c. An analysis of the effect of therapeutic touch on patients' anxiety levels _____

_____

d. An analysis of the effect of depression on students' attrition from a nursing program _____

_____

9. In the following examples, which multivariate procedure is most appropriate for analyzing the data?

a. A researcher is testing the effect of verbal expressiveness, self-esteem, age, and the availability of family supports among a group of recently discharged psychiatric patients on recidivism (*i.e.*, whether they will be readmitted within 12 months after discharge). _____

_____

b. A researcher is comparing the bereavement and coping processes of recently widowed and divorced individuals, controlling for their age.

_____

_____

c. A researcher wants to test the effects of two drug treatments and two dosages of each drug on blood pressure and on the pH and PO_2 levels of arterial blood gases. _____

_____

d. A researcher wants to predict hospital staff absentee rates (number of days absent) based on staff rank, shift, number of years with the hospital, and marital status. _____

_____

10. Below is a list of variables that a nurse researcher might be interested in predicting. For each, suggest at least three independent variables that could be used in a multiple regression analysis.

a. Leadership in nursing supervisors _____

_____

b. Nurses' frequency of administering pain medication _____

_____

c. Proficiency in doing patient interviews _____

_____

d. Patient satisfaction with nursing care _____

_____

e. Anxiety levels of prostatectomy patients _____

_____

■ D. Application Exercises

1. Below is a brief description of a fictitious study, followed by a critique. Do you agree with the critique? Can you add other comments relevant to issues discussed in Chapter 13 of the textbook? (Box 13-2 offers some guiding questions.)

Fictitious Study. Lawton (2001) studied psychological distress and marital satisfaction in a sample of infertile and sterile couples. He hypothesized that levels of well-being and satisfaction would be related to whether the source of the fertility problem was the person him- or herself or the person's partner. He also hypothesized that, overall, women would be more adversely affected than men by the fertility problem. Lawton's sample consisted of 100 couples who were patients at an infertility clinic—50 couples for whom infertility had been diagnosed as attributable to male factors and 50 for whom infertility was attributable to female factors.

Table 13-A is Lawton's table summarizing the demographic characteristics of the four groups of subjects. Lawton administered a questionnaire to all 200 subjects. The questionnaire included 45 Likert-type questions, which Lawton used to create three psychological scales, labeled as follows: (1) depression, (2) marital satisfaction, and (3) feelings of gender-role inadequacy. The scores on the

Table 13-A   Major Characteristics of the Research Sample

| Characteristic | Personal Infertility | | | | Partner Infertility | | | |
| | Males | | Females | | Males | | Females | |
	$\bar{X}$	SD	$\bar{X}$	SD	$\bar{X}$	SD	$\bar{X}$	SD
Age	28.7	3.2	29.8	5.4	30.2	4.6	25.4	2.8
Number of years of education	13.2	1.7	11.8	1.3	13.6	2.0	12.0	1.5
Number of children	.2	.1	.1	.1	.7	.3	.4	.2
Number of years married	5.2	1.3	4.2	.9	4.2	.9	5.2	1.3
Number of subjects	50		50		50		50	

three scales were analyzed in three separate two-way (2 × 2) ANOVAs, with gender and source of the fertility problem as the independent variables. Table 13-B summarizes the results of Lawton's analyses. Lawton concluded on the basis of these data that his hypotheses were partially supported.

Table 13-B   Summary of Analysis of Variance Results

| Dependent Variable | Source of Fertility Problem | Mean Scores | | F-Test Results |
		Males	Females	
Depression scale scores	Self	20.1	29.1	Sex: $F = 5.9, p < .05$
	Partner	15.3	23.6	Source: $F = 6.7, p < .01$
				Sex × Source: $F = 1.9$, NS
Marital satisfaction scale scores	Self	25.6	26.3	Sex: $F = 1.1$, NS
	Partner	28.7	24.9	Source: $F = 0.9$, NS
				Sex × Source: $F = 1.3$, NS
Sex role inadequacy scale scores	Self	27.5	38.9	Sex: $F = 6.4, p < .05$
	Partner	19.5	22.8	Source: $F = 9.3, p < .01$
				Sex × Source: $F = 4.9, p < .05$

Critique. Lawton used Table 13-A to present some basic background information about the four groups of subjects in his study. The table specifies for each group the mean and standard deviation for four variables that were not used in testing the research hypotheses but that provide the reader with a picture of the subjects. The mean and standard deviation appear to be the appropriate indexes for most of the characteristics, although the use of percentages would probably have been more illuminating in the case of the variable *number of children.* For example, it would have been more useful to know that 10% of the men with a fertility problem had previously fathered a child. The mean value of .2 children could be distorted because some of the men may have fathered several children, while most may have never been a parent. The columns and rows in Table 13-A are clearly labeled so that we can look up a piece of information fairly easily. For example, the mean age of women who had a fertility problem was 29.8, while the mean age of women whose partners had a fertility problem was 25.4. Although the layout of the table is acceptable as presented, the reader might have found it easier to interpret the information if the groups had been reordered so that the male and female partners in a couple were in adjacent columns. In the present version, the males in the first column are married to the females in the fourth column, so that the format makes it difficult to understand *couple* characteristics.

Lawton used inferential statistics to test his research hypotheses and succinctly summarized a considerable amount of information about the results in Table 13-B. The table tells us the mean scale scores for the three dependent variables for all four groups of subjects. Standard deviations were not presented, but it is possible that there were few group differences in variability and that the overall standard deviations were therefore reported in the text of the research report. The table also tells us the value of the *F* statistic and the level of significance of the test for both the main and interaction effects. Degrees of freedom are not specified, presumably because they were the same for all tests.

Lawton's choice of a two-way ANOVA seems fairly well suited to his research design, hypotheses, and measures. His design called for the collection of data from both partners of 100 couples, half of whom were diagnosed as having a male-based fertility problem, and the other half a female-based problem. His hypotheses involved both the gender-of-subject factor and a source-of-problem factor. His measures involved two nominal-level independent variables (gender and source of problem) and interval-level dependent variables (the scale scores). The use of a parametric procedure seems justified, although if we had more information about the distribution of the scale scores we might learn that the distributions were too skewed to warrant parametric statistical tests.

Lawton did not use any multivariate statistics, but he might well have done so. For example, there is no indication that factor analysis was used to analyze the underlying dimensionality of the 45 Likert items. The scales were apparently created based on the researcher's judgment. Such judgments are frequently erroneous, however. A factor analysis might have revealed that there were really four (or more) important dimensions being tapped by the 45 Likert statements. The use of four rather than three dependent variables could alter the nature of the researcher's findings and conclusions. Other multivariate procedures might also have been appropriate. For example, ANCOVA could have been used to control such extraneous variables as age, socioeconomic status, and parenting history of the subjects. Table 13-A suggests, for example, that there was some variability among the four groups in terms of these characteristics. Controlling them could alter the findings and lead to different conclusions about the relationship between the independent variables and the dependent variables.

The results of Lawton's study indicated that the women were significantly more depressed and felt less adequate about their gender roles than their husbands (regardless of the source of the fertility problem), consistent with his hypothesis. Also as hypothesized, the person who was the source of the fertility problem was more depressed and had greater feelings of gender-role inadequacy than the person's partner (regardless of gender). Differences relating to marital satisfaction were not statistically significant; the observed differences on this scale were probably the result of random fluctuations only. Thus, Lawton's hypothesis regarding marital satisfaction was not supported by the data.

Although not specifically hypothesized, there was one more significant effect: On the gender-role inadequacy scale, the interaction between gender and source of the problem was significant at the .05 level. An inspection of the means reveals that this interaction does not involve a crossover effect. In the example shown in Table 13-11 of the textbook, it may be recalled, an interaction was observed: Freshmen students had higher test scores when exposed to the lecture, while sophomore students had higher test scores when exposed to the film. In Lawton's data, the interaction is somewhat different. We can interpret the results as follows: Overall, the women had more negative gender-role feelings than the men; overall, the people who were the source of the fertility problem felt worse about gender-role inadequacy than those whose partners were the source; *but* being a woman *and* being the source of the fertility problem had a compounding effect that resulted in the highest scores on the gender-role inadequacy scale.

Note that because this is an ex post facto study, there is nothing in the data to establish causal relationships. Lawton cannot conclude that depression and feelings of gender-role inadequacy are a consequence of an infertility problem or of being the responsible party in a couple's fertility problem. The direction of causality, after all, might be reversed: People who are depressed may have a psychogenic block that inhibits fertility. Or, the results could reflect the effects of some other characteristics that differentiate the four groups. Statistical significance tells us nothing about whether there is a cause-and-effect relationship; it tells us that there is a high probability that the relation exists in the population.

2. Here is a brief summary of another fictitious study. Read the summary and then respond to the questions that follow.

Mouzon (2000) hypothesized that infants' sleeping problems were related to various conditions and experiences during their birth. Fifty infants aged 3 to 6 months were diagnosed as having severe sleep-disturbance problems. A group of 50 infants aged 3 to 6 months who had normal sleeping patterns was used as the comparison group. Mouzon obtained the hospital records for all 100 children. The two groups were compared in terms of the following variables: amount of anesthesia administered during labor and delivery (none, small amount, large amount); length of time in labor (number of hours and minutes); type of delivery (cesarean or vaginal); birth weight (in grams); and Apgar scores at 3 minutes (scores from 1 to 10). Mouzon found that the sleep-disturbance group had

had significantly longer time in labor than the comparison group. The groups were comparable in terms of the other variables.

Review and critique this research effort. Suggest alternative measurement approaches. To assist you in your critique, here are some guiding questions.

   a. How many variables were measured in this study?
   b. For each variable, identify the level of measurement that was used.
   c. For each variable, indicate whether the measurement could have been made at a higher level of measurement than the level that was used. If yes, specify how you might measure the variable to obtain a higher level measure.
   d. For two of the variables, write out operational definitions that clearly indicate the rules of measurement for those variables.

3. Below are several suggested research articles. Read one of these articles, paying special attention to the ways in which the research variables were operationalized. Evaluate the researcher's measurement strategy, using parts **a** to **d** of Question D.2 as a guide.

   ■ Barnfather, J. S., & Ronis, D. L. (2000). Test of a model of psychosocial resources, stress, and health among undereducated adults. *Research in Nursing & Health, 23,* 55–66.

   ■ Lipman, T. H., Hayman, L. L., Fabian, C. V., DiFazio, D. A., Hale, P. M., Goldsmith, B. M., & Piascik, P. C. (2000). Risk factors for cardiovascular disease in children with Type I diabetes. *Nursing Research, 49,* 160–166.

   ■ MacMullen, N. J., & Dulski, L. A. (2000). Factors related to sucking ability in healthy newborns. *Journal of Obstetric, Gynecologic, and Neonatal Nursing, 29,* 390–396.

   ■ Stark, M. A. (2000). Is it difficult to concentrate during the third trimester and postpartum? *Journal of Obstetric, Gynecologic, and Neonatal Nursing, 29,* 378–389.

4. Here is another brief summary of a fictitious study. Read the summary and then respond to the questions that follow.

Balmuth (2000) hypothesized that patients with a high degree of physical mobility would describe themselves as being healthier than patients with less physical mobility. To test this hypothesis, 120 male patients in a Veterans Administration hospital were asked to rate themselves on a 5-point scale regarding their current physical health (1 = very unhealthy and 5 = very healthy) and to predict the number of days that they would be hospitalized. Forty of these patients had been categorized as "of limited mobility," another 40 were classified as "of moderate mobility," and the remaining 40 were described as "of high mobility." Balmuth reported his descriptive findings as follows:

> The self-ratings of physical health were fairly normally distributed for the sample as a whole: 42% rated themselves as neither healthy nor unhealthy; 7% and 21% described themselves as "very healthy" or "somewhat healthy," respectively. At the other extreme, 6% said they were "very unhealthy," and 24% said "somewhat unhealthy." The three groups differed in this regard, however. In the high-mobility group, a full 45% said they were either "very" or "somewhat healthy," while only 30% of the moderate-mobility and 15% of the low-mobility groups said this. For the entire sample, the mean predicted length of stay was 14.1 days. The median length, however, was only 12.5 days. For the three groups, the means and standard deviations with respect to predicted length of stay in hospital were as follows:

	Mean	Standard Deviation
High Mobility	7.1	3.2
Moderate Mobility	11.9	4.5
Low Mobility	23.3	7.4

> In this sample of patients, the correlation between predicted length of stay in hospital and the health rating was .56.

Review and critique this study, particularly with respect to the statistical analysis. To assist you in this critique, here are some guiding questions.

a. Which of the following types of descriptive statistical methods were used in this example?
   Frequency distribution
   Measure of central tendency
   Measure of variability
   Contingency table
   Correlation
b. Comment on the appropriateness of each statistic reported in the example. Is the statistic appropriate given the level of measurement of the variable? Does the statistic throw away information? Is the statistic the most stable statistic possible?

c. Identify two or three statistics that were not reported by the researcher that *could* have been reported, given the data that were collected. Evaluate the extent to which the absence of this information weakened (or streamlined) the report of the results.

d. Discuss the meaning of the means and standard deviations in this example.

5. Below are several suggested research articles. Skim one (or more) of these articles and respond to parts **a** to **d** of Question D.4 in terms of the actual research study. (At this point, ignore the references to tests of statistical significance, which are covered in subsequent exercises.)

■ Bungum, T. J., Peaslee, D.L., Jackson, A.W., & Perez, M.A. (2000). Exercise during pregnancy and type of delivery in nulliparae. *Journal of Obstetric, Gynecologic, and Neonatal Nursing, 29,* 258–264.

■ Courts, N.F. (2000). Psychosocial adjustment of patients on home hemodialysis and their dialysis partners. *Clinical Nursing Research, 9,* 177–190.

■ Marinella, M.A., Kathula, S.K., & Markert, R.J. (2000). Spectrum of upper-extremity deep venous thrombosis in a community teaching hospital. *Heart & Lung, 29,* 113–117.

■ McClanahan, P., & Edwards, M.R. (2000). Characteristics of Norplant users. *Journal of Obstetric, Gynecologic, and Neonatal Nursing, 29,* 275–281.

6. Below is another brief summary of a fictitious study. Read the summary and then respond to the questions that follow.

Curtis (2001) investigated whether taste acuity declines with age, using a cross-sectional design. Eighty subjects were given a taste acuity test in which they were asked to indicate, for 25 substances, whether the taste was salty, sweet, bitter, or sour. The substances were presented in randomized order. Each person had five scores: four scores corresponding to the correct identification of the substances in the four taste categories, and one total score. Twenty subjects from each of the following age groups were tested: 31 to 40; 41 to 50; 51 to 60; and 61 to 70 years. It was hypothesized that taste acuity would decline with age, both overall and for all four subcategories of taste. The mean test scores for the four groups on all five outcomes measures appear below, together with information on the statistical tests performed.

	Age Group						
	31–40	41–50	51–60	61–70	F	df	p
Salty test	6.3	5.8	5.7	5.4	3.5	3,76	<.05
Sweet test	5.0	5.0	5.4	5.2	1.2	3,76	>.05
Bitter test	4.0	4.1	3.7	3.3	2.6	3,76	>.05
Sour test	1.9	2.0	2.0	2.1	0.8	3,76	>.05
Overall test	17.2	16.9	16.8	16.0	2.4	3,76	>.05

Curtis concluded that her hypothesis was only partially supported by the data.

Review and critique the above study. Suggest possible alternatives for handling the analysis of the data. To assist you in your critique, here are some guiding questions.

a. For each of the variables, indicate the actual level of measurement as used, then indicate the highest possible level of measurement for each. Is there a discrepancy? If so, can you think of a justification for it?
b. What statistical test was used to analyze the data? Did the researcher use the appropriate statistical test? If not, what statistical test do you think would be more suitable?
c. Are the degrees of freedom as presented correct?
d. Which of the results is statistically significant—that is, which hypothesis was supported by the data? Describe the meaning of each of the statistical tests.

7. Below are several suggested research articles. Skim one (or more) of these articles and respond to parts **a** to **d** of Question D.6 in terms of the actual research study.

   ■ King, K. B., Rowe, M. A., & Zerwic, J. J. (2000). Concerns and risk factor modification in women during the year after coronary artery surgery. *Nursing Research, 49*, 167–172.

   ■ Koniak-Griffin, D., Anderson, N., Verzemnieks, I., & Brecht, M. (2000). A public health nursing early intervention program for adolescent mothers. *Nursing Research, 49*, 130–138,

   ■ Moser, D. K., Dracup, K., & Doering, L. V. (2000). Factors differentiating dropouts from completers in a longitudinal, multicenter clinical trial. *Nursing Research, 49*, 109–116.

   ■ Schmelzer, M., Case, P., Chappell, S. M., & Wright, K. B. (2000). Colonic cleansing, fluid absorption, and discomfort following tap water and soapsuds enemas. *Applied Nursing Research, 13*, 83–91.

■ E. Special Projects

1. Fictitious data from 24 nurses for six variables are presented below. Compute and present five to ten different descriptive statistics that you think would best summarize this information.

Subject No.	Shift[a]	Anxiety Scores[b]	Supervisor's Performance Rating[c]	No. of Years of Experience	Marital Status[d]	Job Satisfaction Score[e]
1	1	10	4	5	2	4
2	1	13	4	2	2	5
3	1	8	2	1	1	3
4	1	4	7	10	1	3
5	1	6	9	12	1	4
6	1	9	8	7	1	2
7	1	12	6	8	2	4
8	1	5	4	2	1	5
9	2	10	5	4	2	1
10	2	14	6	1	2	4
11	2	8	5	3	1	5
12	2	15	8	2	2	2
13	2	11	8	7	2	3
14	2	14	7	9	1	1
15	2	1	5	3	2	2
16	2	8	8	6	1	3
17	3	3	7	19	2	4
18	3	7	4	7	1	1
19	3	19	5	1	2	2
20	3	5	6	11	1	1
21	3	8	3	2	1	3
22	3	10	4	5	2	2
23	3	13	6	6	2	1
24	3	14	5	3	1	2

[a]1 = day; 2 = evening; 3 = night
[b]Scores are from a low of 0 to a high of 20; 20 = most anxious
[c]Ratings are from 1 = poor to 9 = excellent
[d]1 = married; 2 = not married
[e]Scores are from low of 1 to high of 5; 5 = most satisfied

2. Ask 20 friends, classmates, or colleagues the following three questions:

   ■ How many brothers and sisters do you have?

   ■ How many children do you expect to have in total?

   ■ Would you describe your family during your childhood as "very close," "fairly close," or "not very close"?

   When you have gathered your data, calculate and present several statistics that describe the information you obtained.

3. Below is a list of variables. Assume that you have data from 500 nurses on these variables. Develop two or three hypotheses regarding the relationships among these variables and indicate what statistical tests you would use to test your hypotheses.

   ■ Number of years of nursing experience

   ■ Type of employment setting (hospital, nursing school, public school system, etc.)

   ■ Salary

   ■ Marital status

   ■ Job satisfaction ("dissatisfied," "neither dissatisfied nor satisfied," or "satisfied")

   ■ Number of children under age 18

   ■ Gender

4. Design and describe a study in which you would use both factor analysis and ANCOVA.

CHAPTER **14**

Analyzing Qualitative Data

■ A. Matching Exercises

1. Match each descriptive statement from Set B with one of the types of analytic strategy from Set A. Indicate the letter corresponding to your response next to each item in Set B.

SET A

a. Quasi-statistical style

b. Template analysis style

c. Editing analysis style

d. Immersion/crystallization style

SET B	RESPONSES
1. Approach is sometimes referred to as manifest content analysis.	_____
2. Researcher becomes totally involved in and reflective of the data.	_____
3. Grounded theory approach typically adopts this analytic style.	_____
4. Fits the data to a pre-conceived codebook or category scheme.	_____
5. Type of style most likely to be adopted by ethnographers.	_____
6. Researcher develops an analysis guide that is used to sort and interpret the data.	_____

■ B. Completion Exercises

Write the words or phrases that correctly complete the sentences below.

1. Data collection and data analysis typically occur _____ _____ in qualitative studies, not as separate phases.

2. The four processes that play a role in qualitative analysis are _____, _____, _____, and _____.

3. The main task in organizing qualitative data involves the development of a method of _____ and _____ the data.

4. The process of breaking down the data, examining them, and comparing them to other segments is referred to as _____.

5. In a grounded theory study, the initial phase of coding is referred to as _____.

6. A _____ is a physical file that is organized to contain all material relating to a topic area.

7. Traditional methods of organizing qualitative data are being replaced by _____.

8. The analysis of qualitative data generally begins with a search for _____.

9. The use of _____ involves an accounting of the frequency with which certain themes and relationships are supported by the data.

10. In grounded theory studies, coding of information relating only to the core variable is referred to as _____coding.

11. A particular type of core variable in a grounded theory study is the _____ or BSP.

12. Colaizzi, Giorgi, and VanKaam's methods of analysis are used to analyze data from a study within the _____ tradition.

13. One of VanManen's approaches to data analysis is referred to as the _____ approach, which involves an analysis of every sentence of data.

■ C. Study Questions

1. Define the following terms. Compare your definition with the definition in Chapter 14 of the textbook or in the glossary.

   a. Qualitative analysis _____

   _____

   b. Open coding _____

   _____

   c. Categorization scheme _____

   _____

   d. Template _____

   _____

   e. Theme _____

   _____

   f. Conceptual file _____

   _____

   g. Memo _____

   _____

   h. Selective coding _____

   _____

   i. Core variable _____

   _____

   j. Duquesne school _____

   _____

   k. Utrecht school _____

   _____

2. For each of the research questions below, indicate whether you think a researcher should collect primarily qualitative or quantitative data. Justify your response.

a. How do victims of AIDS cope with the discovery of their illness?

_____

_____

b. What important dimensions of nursing practice differ in developed and underdeveloped countries? _____

_____

c. What is the effect of therapeutic touch on patient well-being?

_____

_____

d. Do nurse practitioners and physicians differ in the performance of triage functions? _____

_____

e. Is a patient's length of stay in hospital related to the quality or quantity of his or her social supports? _____

_____

f. How does the typical American feel about such new reproductive technologies as in vitro fertilization? _____

_____

g. What are the psychological sequelae of having an organ transplantation? _____

_____

h. By what processes do women make decisions about having amniocentesis? _____

_____

i. What factors are most predictive of a woman giving birth to a very-low-birthweight infant? _____

_____

j. What effects does caffeine have on gastrointestinal motility?

_____

_____

3. A category scheme for coding interviews with recently divorced women follows:
   1. Divorce-related issues
      a. Adjustment to divorce
      b. Divorce-induced problems
      c. Advantages of divorce
   2. General psychologic state
      a. Before divorce
      b. During divorce
      c. Current
   3. Physical health
      a. Before divorce
      b. During divorce
      c. Current
   4. Relationship with children
      a. General quality
      b. Communication
      c. Shared activities
      d. Structure of relationship
   5. Parenting
      a. Discipline and child-rearing
      b. Feelings about parenthood
      c. Feelings about single parenthood
   6. Friendships/social participation
      a. Dating and marriage
      b. Friendships
      c. Social groups, leisure
      d. Social support
   7. Employment/Education
      a. Employment experiences
      b. Education experiences
      c. Job and career goals
      d. Educational goals
   8. Workload
      a. Coping with workload
      b. Schedule
      c. Child care arrangements
   9. Finances

Read the following excerpt, taken from a real interview. Use the coding scheme to code the topics discussed in this excerpt using the margins to write in codes.

> I think raising the children is so much easier without the father around. There isn't two people conflicting back and forth. You know, like . . . like you discipline them during the day. They do something wrong,

you're not saying, "When daddy gets home, you're going to get a spanking." You know, you do that. The kid gets a spanking right then and there. But when two people live together, they have their ways of raising and you have your ways of raising the children and it's so hard for two people to raise children. It's so much easier for one person. The only reason a male would be around is financial-wise. But me and the kids are happier now, and we get along with each other better, cause like, there isn't this competitive thing. My husband always wanted all the attention around here.

■ D. Application Exercises

1. Below is a brief description of the data analysis in a fictitious qualitative study, followed by a critique. Do you agree with this critique? Can you add other comments relevant to the data analysis in this study? (Box 14-1 offers some guiding questions.)

Fictitious Study. VanMeter (2000) was interested in learning about the health policies and health environments of child care centers. She began her study by spending a week in an urban day care center that provided child care services to children aged 10 weeks to preschool-age. The purpose of this preliminary step was to ascertain sources of information and to familiarize herself with the routine of child care environments.

The data for the study were collected through unstructured interviews with child care staff, through observation of activities during normal operating hours, and through the gathering of formal health policy statements from the administrators of the centers. The interviews with the staff focused on how staff handled illnesses among the children, what the patterns of illnesses were, how parents were notified in the case of a midday illness, to what extent medications were administered by the staff, and how the staff interpreted center policies relating to the admission of unwell children. Data were collected from 10 child care centers that served 25 or more children whose ages ranged from infant to preschool-age. A total of 68 staff interviews were completed.

VanMeter's field notes from the observations and the interviews were transcribed and coded according to a coding scheme that evolved during the actual collection of data. Three major themes emerged from the data analysis. These were labeled *uncertainty, conflict,* and *frustration.* The types of evidence that gave rise to the uncertainty category included statements made by staff, such as: "I'm really not a very good judge of just where to draw the line in deciding whether to keep a child here or send her home"; "I can't really remember what our health policies say on that"; and "I don't really know what the major health problems are among our kids—when they're absent, I just have one less kid to worry about."

Evidence of the conflict dimension included the researcher's observation that staff and parents sometimes had disagreements about whether a child was not well enough to attend. Also, staff made such statements as: "Health is a problem in child care centers because, on the one hand, allowing a sick kid to attend means that we'll have a lot of sick kids, but on the other hand, it's really tough on parents when their child care arrangements fall apart."

The category of frustration emerged from such statements as: "It's difficult to plan activities because absenteeism for health reasons is such a problem right now" and "I can't seem to get the kids interested in thinking about good health or good nutrition—their parents are just as bad."

VanMeter analyzed the data herself but shared preliminary results of her analyses with one of the directors of a child care center, who concurred with the thematic analysis. VanMeter's analysis revealed that centers that had a formal arrangement with a health care provider were less likely to have staff who were uncertain. Conflict was a fairly universal theme but appeared to be more prevalent among those centers that served predominantly low-income families. Frustration was most likely to be observed and expressed among staff caring for older children.

Critique. Given VanMeter's broad area of interest in health issues within child care centers, it seems appropriate that she conducted an in-depth, multifaceted qualitative study. The use of three complementary sources of data strengthened her study because it provided an opportunity for validating findings. At least from the brief description presented, however, it does not appear that these data sources were fully exploited. For example, no use appears to have been made of the written policy statements.

It appears that the author did little to validate the subjective thematic analysis. The analysis would have been greatly strengthened if VanMeter had involved another investigator in the coding and analysis, if she had systematically searched for contrary evidence regarding the important themes, or if there had been an iterative approach in the analysis to check emerging themes against the data. Although it is laudable that VanMeter invited comments from one of the child care center's directors, this procedure by itself provided a relatively weak form of validation.

The true validity of VanMeter's thematic analysis is difficult to evaluate thoroughly without actually inspecting the data, but the brief description does not provide persuasive evidence that the analysis was thorough and unbiased. The data sources should have yielded a wealth of information about various aspects of the health policies and practices of the day care centers. Yet all three themes focus on the staff's *feelings*, and in all three cases these are negative feelings. What about their actions? What about their levels of competence in dealing with health issues? What about their sensitivity to the needs of their clients? It would appear that several of the excerpts included in support of VanMeter's thematic analysis could have been conceptualized in a different way, suggesting that perhaps VanMeter had some preconceived notions about what the unstructured interviews and observations would yield. It is possible that a reconceptualization (i.e., a thematic analysis of the same materials by a different investigator) could completely alter our impression of the health practices and policies of child care centers.

2. Here is a brief summary of another fictitious qualitative study. Read the summary and then respond to the questions that follow.

DelSette (2001) studied the phenomenon of "being on precautions" from the perspective of hospitalized adults. She began her study, after securing authorization, by spending two days on the hospital units where the data would be collected. The two days were spent familiarizing herself with the units, learning how best to collect the data, determining where she could position herself in an unobtrusive manner, and establishing a trusting relationship with the nursing staff.

The data for the study were collected using the techniques of observation and unstructured interviewing. DelSette selectively sampled all times of the day and all days of the week in 2-hour segments to make her observations. The time schedule began on a Monday morning at 7:00 AM and continued until 9:00 AM. On Tuesday, the observation time became 9:00 AM until 11:00 AM. Observations continued around the clock on consecutive days until no new information was being collected. DelSette either positioned herself directly outside the door to the patient's room or sat in the patient's room to make her observations. Observations included any activity or interaction between the patient and hospital staff or between the patient and DelSette. The unstructured interviewing process consisted of asking patients to clarify why they were doing certain things and what they liked or disliked about the hospital experience.

DelSette recorded the observations and data from the interviews in a log immediately after each 2-hour observation segment. All data were recorded in chronologic order. DelSette also recorded any feelings she had during the observation experience. As time progressed, she reread her field notes after every 4 hours of observation. As commonalities began to emerge from the data, she developed another section to her log according to similarity of content and referenced the daily log notes according to commonalities. DelSette continued making observations until she thought she had a "good feel for the data" and that additional observations or interactions would provide only redundant information. A total of five patients were observed.

Categories that emerged from the data were labeled "avoidance," "devaluation as a person," and "loneliness." Evidence for the avoidance perspective came from patient comments during informal conversations with the researcher and the observational field notes. The evidence included statements such as, "Nurses seldom come into the room because they have to put all that [pointing to precaution gowns] stuff on"; "Look, she [the cleaning woman] won't come in the room. She's afraid of me"; "Did you see that? Only my doctor would touch me. The rest were afraid to touch me." Observational field notes contained several notations of nurses coming to the door of the room asking, "Do you want anything?" but not entering the room.

The category "devaluation as a person" emerged from comments such as, "I don't like being treated as a specimen"; "Do you have to wear gloves every time you take care of me [made to a nurse]?"; "If I go to the door of the room, they [the nurses] yell at me [made to the researcher]."

The category "loneliness" was developed from field notes that observed patients occasionally putting the call light on to find out what time it was or how long until lunch, or asking about a noise they had heard. Comments that conveyed the same feeling of loneliness were, "Being confined in this room is like being in jail"; "I can't wait to get out of here and have dinner with my friends"; and "The hours seem endless here."

Review and critique this study. Suggest alternative ways of collecting and analyzing the data for the research problem. To assist you in your critique, here are some guiding questions:

   a. Comment on the choice of research approach. Was a qualitative research approach suitable for the phenomenon being studied? In your opinion, would a more quantitative research approach have been more appropriate?
   b. The data in the study were collected by observation and informal interviewing. Could the data have been collected in another way? Should they have been?
   c. What type of sampling plan was used to sample observations in the study? Would an alternative sampling plan have been better? Why or why not?
   d. The researcher recorded her observations, feelings, and interviews immediately after each 2-hour observation period. Comment on the appropriateness of this method. Can you identify any biases that could be present in this choice of method? Suggest alternative ways of recording the data.
   e. Categorize the field notes made in the study according to their purpose. What additional types of field notes would you have included?
   f. How did the researcher handle the concept of theoretical saturation? Could you recommend any improvements?
   g. What types of validation procedures did the researcher use? Can you suggest additional procedures that might have improved the study?
   h. Comment on the categories that emerged from the data. Do they appear to reflect accurately the data that were collected? Would you have developed different ones?

2. Below are several suggested research articles. Skim one or more of these articles and respond to questions a through h from Question D.2, to the extent possible, in terms of the actual research study.

   ■ Carolan, M. (2000). Menopause: Irish women's voices. *Journal of Obstetric, Gynecologic, and Neonatal Nursing, 29,* 397–404.

- Lock, S. E., Ferguson, S. L., & Wise, C. (1998). Communication of sexual risk behavior among late adolescents. *Western Journal of Nursing Research, 20,* 273–294.

- Porter, E. J., Ganong, L. H., & Armer, J. M. (2000). The church family and kin: An older rural black woman's support network and preferences for care providers. *Qualitative Health Research, 10,* 452–470.

- Rush, K. L., & Ouellet, L. L. (1998). An analysis of elderly clients' view of mobility. *Western Journal of Nursing Research, 20,* 295–311.

- Torsch, V. L., & Ma, G. X. (2000). Cross-cultural comparison of health perceptions, concerns, and coping strategies among Asian and Pacific Islander American elders. *Qualitative Health Research, 10,* 471–489.

■ E. Special Projects

1. Get ten or so people to write one or two paragraphs on their feelings about death and dying. Perform a thematic analysis of these paragraphs.

2. Develop two or three research questions that you think might lend themselves to a qualitative study.

3. Read one of the studies listed in the Suggested Readings section of Chapter 14 in the textbook. Generate several hypotheses that could be tested based on the reported findings.

PART VI

Critical Appraisal and Utilization of Nursing Research

CHAPTER 15

Critiquing Research Reports

■ A. Matching Exercises

1. Match each of the questions in Set B with the research decision for quantitative studies that is being evaluated, as listed in Set A. Indicate the letter corresponding to your response next to each of the statements in Set B.

SET A

a. Research design decisions
b. The population and sampling plan
c. Data collection procedures
d. Analytic decisions

SET B   RESPONSES

1. Was there a sufficient number of subjects?   _____

2. Was there evidence of adequate reliability and validity?   _____

3. Would a more limited specification have controlled some
   extraneous variables not covered by the research design?   _____

4. Would nonparametric tests have been more appropriate?   _____

5. Should a stratified design have been used?   _____

6. Were threats to internal validity adequately controlled?   _____

7. Were the statistical tests appropriate, given the level of
   measurement of the variables?   _____

8. Were response set biases minimized?   _____

9. Was the comparison group equivalent to the experimental
   group?   _____

10. Should the data have been collected prospectively?   _____

2. Match each of the questions in Set B with the research decision for qualitative studies that is being evaluated, as listed in Set A. Indicate the letter corresponding to your response next to each of the statements in Set B.

SET A

a. The setting
b. Data sources and data quality
c. Sampling plan
d. Data analysis

SET B   **RESPONSES**

1. Were triangulation procedures used as a method of validation?   _____

2. Were there a sufficient number of study participants to achieve saturation?   _____

3. Were constant comparison procedures appropriately used to refine relevant categories?   _____

4. Was the method of data collection appropriate and sufficient?   _____

5. Were participants asked to comment on the emerging themes?   _____

6. Did the study take place in an information-rich location?   _____

7. Were the study participants the best possible informants?   _____

8. Do the themes seem parsimonious, logical, and non-superficial?   _____

■ B. Completion Exercises

1. The first step in the interpretation of research findings involves an analysis of the _____ of the results, based on various types of evidence.

2. Interpretation of quantitative results is easiest when the results are consistent with the researcher's _____.

3. An important research precept is that correlation does not prove _____.

4. Researchers should avoid the temptation of going beyond _____ _____.

5. Statistical significance does not necessarily mean that research results are
   _____.

6. The research process involves numerous methodologic _____
   _____, each of which could affect the quality of the
   study.

7. A good critique should identify both _____
   and _____ in a study.

8. An evaluation of the relevance of a study to some aspect of the nursing
   profession involves critiquing the _____
   dimension of a research study.

9. An evaluation of the researcher's study design involves critiquing the
   _____ dimension of a research study.

10. An evaluation of the way in which human subjects were treated involves
    critiquing the _____ dimension of a research study.

11. An evaluation of the sense the researcher tried to make of the results in-
    volves critiquing the _____ dimen-
    sion of the research study.

12. An evaluation of the conciseness and organization of the research report
    involves critiquing the _____
    dimension of the research study.

■ C. Study Questions

1. Define the following terms. Use the textbook to compare your definitions
   with the definitions in Chapter 15 or in the Glossary.

   a. Critique _____
   _____

   b. Results _____
   _____

   c. Interpretation of results _____
   _____

   d. Unhypothesized results _____
   _____

   e. Mixed results _____
   _____

2. Read and critique one or more of the following research reports (or others in the nursing research literature). Prepare two or three pages of "bullet points" that indicate the major strengths and weaknesses of the study.

Quantitative Studies

- Badger, T. A., & Collins-Joyce, P. (2000). Depression, psychosocial resources, and functional ability in older adults. *Clinical Nursing Research, 9,* 238–255.

- Connelly, B., Gunzerath, L., & Knebel, A. (2000). A pilot study exploring mood state and dyspnea in mechanically ventilated patients. *Heart & Lung, 29,* 173–179.

- McCarthy, D. O. (2000). Tumor necrosis factor alpha and interleukin-6 have differential effects on food intake and gastric emptying in fasted rats. *Research in Nursing & Health, 23,* 222–228.

- Neu, M., Browne, J. V., & Vojir, C. (2000). The impact of two transfer techniques used during skin-to-skin care on the physiologic and behavioral responses of preterm infants. *Nursing Research, 49,* 215–223.

- Watt-Watson, J., Garfinkel, P., Gallop, R., Stevens, B., & Streiner, D. (2000). The impact of nurses' empathic responses on patients' pain management in acute care. *Nursing Research, 49,* 191–200.

Qualitative Studies

- Chiu, L. (2000). Lived experience of spirituality in Taiwanese women with breast cancer. *Western Journal of Nursing Research, 22,* 29–53.

- Hilton, B. A., Crawford, J. A., & Tarko, M. A. (2000). Men's perspectives on individual and family coping with their wives' breast cancer and chemotherapy. *Western Journal of Nursing Research, 22,* 438–459.

- Schirm, V., Albanese, T., Garland, T. N., Gipson, G., & Blackmon, D. J. (2000). Caregiving in nursing homes. *Clinical Nursing Research, 9,* 280–297.

- Schumacher, K. L., Stewart, B. J., Archbold, P. G., Dodd, M. J., & Dibble, S. L. (2000). Family caregiving skill: Development of the concept. *Research in Nursing & Health, 23,* 191–203.

- Wilson, K., & Williams, A. (2000). Visualism in community nursing: Implications for telephone work with service users. *Qualitative Health Research, 10,* 507–520.

3. Read the following qualitative research report and identify the study's major strengths and limitations:

■ Lock, S.E., Ferguson, S. L. & Wise, C. (1998). Communication of sexual risk behavior among late adolescents. *Western Journal of Nursing Research, 20,* 273-289.

Now, read the two commentaries of the study that immediately follow the report (pages 289–294). Do any of your comments overlap with those of the commentators? Do you agree or disagree with either or both sets of comments?

■ D. Application Exercises

1. Below is a fictitious research report and a critique of various aspects of the report. This example is designed to highlight features about the form and content of both a written report and a written evaluation of the study's worth. To economize on space, the report is rather brief, but it incorporates the essential elements for a meaningful appraisal.

    Read the report and critique and then determine whether you agree with the critique. Can you add other comments relevant to a critical appraisal of the study?

The Role of Health Care Providers in Teenage Pregnancy
by Phyllis Nelson, 2000

BACKGROUND

Of the 20 million teenagers living in the United States, about one in four is sexually active by age 14; more than half have had sexual intercourse by age 17 (Kelman and Saner, 1994).[1] Despite increased availability of contraceptives, the number of teenage pregnancies has remained fairly stable over the past two decades. About one million girls under age 20 become pregnant each year and, of these, about 500,000 become teenaged mothers (U.S. Bureau of the Census, 1993).

Public concern regarding teenage pregnancy stems not only from the high rates, but also from the extensive research that has documented the adverse consequences of early parenthood in the health arena. Pregnant teenagers have been found to receive less prenatal

---

[1]All references in this example are fictitious. Although most of the information in this fictitious literature review is based on real studies and is, therefore, accurate.

care (Tremain, 1992), to be more likely to develop toxemia (Schendley, 1991; Waters, 1989), to be more likely to experience prolonged labor (Curran, 1989), to be more likely to have low-birth-weight babies (Tremain, 1992; Beach, 1995), and to be more likely to have babies with low Apgar scores (Beach, 1995) than older mothers. The long-term consequences to the teenaged mothers themselves are also extremely bleak: Teenaged mothers get less schooling, are more likely to be on public assistance, are likely to earn lower wages, and are more likely to get divorced if they marry than their peers who postpone parenthood (Jamail, 1989; North, 1992; Smithfield, 1991).

The one million teenagers who become pregnant each year are caught up in a tough emotional decision—to carry the pregnancy to term and keep the baby, to have an abortion, or to deliver the baby and surrender it for adoption. Despite the widely reported adverse consequences of young parenthood cited above, most young women today are opting for delivery and child-rearing, often out of wedlock (Jaffrey, 1994; Henderson, 1991).

The purpose of this study was to test the effect of a special intervention based in an outpatient clinic of a Chicago hospital on improving the health outcomes of a group of pregnant teenagers. Specifically, it was hypothesized that pregnant teenagers who were in the special program would receive more prenatal care, would be less likely to develop toxemia, would be less likely to have a low-birth-weight baby, would spend fewer hours in labor, would have babies with higher Apgar scores, and would be more likely to use a contraceptive at 6 months postpartum than pregnant teenagers not enrolled in the program.

The theoretical model on which this research was based is an ecologic model of personal behavior (Brandenburg, 1984). A schematic diagram of the ecologic model is presented in Figure 15-A. In this framework, the actions of the person are the focus of attention, but those actions are believed to be a function not only of the person's own characteristics, attitudes, and abilities but also of other influences in their environment. Environmental influences can be differentiated according to their proximal relationship with the target person. Health care workers and institutions are, according to the model, more distant influences than family, peers, and boyfriends. Yet it is assumed that these less immediate forces are real and can

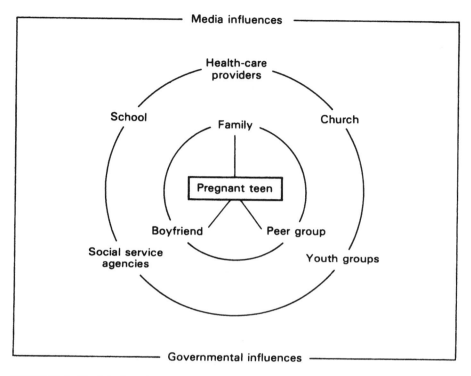

FIGURE 15-A. Model of ecologic contexts

intervene to change the behaviors of the target person. Thus, it is hypothesized that pregnant teenagers can be influenced by increased exposure to a health care team providing a structured program of services designed to promote improved health outcomes.

METHODS

A special program of services for pregnant teenagers was implemented in the outpatient clinic of an inner-city public hospital in Chicago. The intervention involved nutrition education and counseling, parenting education, instruction on prenatal health care, preparation for childbirth, and contraceptive counseling.

All teenagers with a confirmed pregnancy attending the clinic were asked if they wanted to participate in the special program. The goal was to enroll 150 pregnant teenagers during the program's first year of operation. A total of 276 teenagers attending the clinic were invited to participate; of these, 59 had an abortion or miscarriage and 108 declined to participate, yielding an experimental group sample of 109 girls.

To test the effectiveness of the special program, a comparison group of pregnant teenagers was needed. Another inner-city hospital agreed to cooperate in the study. Staff obtained information on the labor and delivery outcomes of the 120 teenagers who delivered at the comparison hospital, where no special teen-parent program was available. For both experimental group and comparison group subjects, a follow-up telephone interview was conducted 6 months postpartum to determine if the teenagers were using birth control.

The independent variable in this study was the teenager's program status: Experimental group members participated in the special program, while comparison group members did not. The dependent variables were the teenagers' labor and delivery and postpartum contraceptive outcomes. The operational definitions of the dependent variables were as follows:

Prenatal care: Number of visits made to a physician or nurse during the pregnancy, exclusive of the visit for the pregnancy test
Toxemia: Presence versus absence of preeclamptic toxemia as diagnosed by a physician
Labor time: Number of hours elapsed from the first contractions until delivery of the baby, to the nearest half hour
Low infant birth weight: Infant birth weights of less than 2500 grams versus those of 2500 grams or greater
Apgar score: Infant Apgar score (from 0 to 10) taken at 3 minutes after birth
Contraceptive use postpartum: Self-reported use of any form of birth control 6 months postpartum versus self-reported nonuse

The two groups were compared on these six outcome measures using *t*-tests and chi-squared tests.

RESULTS

The teenagers in the sample were, on average, 17.6 years old at the time of delivery. The mean age was 17.1 in the experimental group and 18.0 in the comparison group.

By definition, all the teenagers in the experimental group had received prenatal care. Two of the teenagers in the comparison group had no health care treatment before delivery. The distribution of visits for the two groups is presented in Figure 15-B. The experimental group had a higher mean number of prenatal visits than the comparison group, as shown in Table 15-A, but the difference was not statistically significant at the .05 level, using a *t*-test for independent groups.

In the sample as a whole, about 1 girl in 10 was diagnosed as having preeclamptic toxemia. The difference between the two groups was in the hypothesized direction, with 1.6% more of the comparison group teenagers developing this complication, but the difference was not significant using a chi-squared test.

The hours spent in labor ranged from 3.5 to 29.0 in the experimental group and from 4.5 to 33.5 in the comparison group. On average, teenagers in the experimental group spent 14.3 hours in

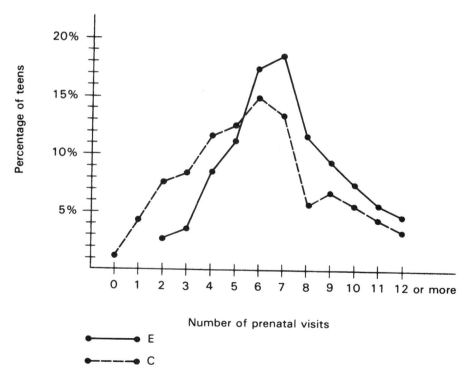

FIGURE 15-B. Frequency distribution of prenatal visits, by experimental versus comparison group. (*E*, experimental group; *C*, comparison group)

Table 15-A Summary of Experimental and Comparison
Group Differences

Outcome Variable	Group		Difference	Test Statistic
	Experimental (n = 109)	Comparison (n = 120)		
Mean number of prenatal visits	7.1	5.9	1.2	$t = 1.83$, $df = 227$, NS
Percentage with toxemia	10.1%	11.7%	−1.6%	$\chi^2 = 0.15$, $df = 1$, NS
Mean hours spent in labor	14.3	15.2	−.09	$t = 1.01$, $df = 227$, NS
Percentage with low-birth-weight baby	16.5%	20.9%	−4.4%	$\chi^2 = 0.71$, $df = 1$, NS
Mean Apgar score	7.3	6.7	.6	$t = 0.98$, $df = 227$, NS
Percentage adopting contraception post-partum	81.7%	62.5%	19.2%	$\chi^2 = 10.22$, $df = 1$, $p < .01$

labor, compared with 15.2 for the comparison group teenagers. The difference was not statistically significant.

With regard to low-birth-weight babies, a total of 43 girls out of 229 in the sample gave birth to babies who weighed under 2500 grams (5.5 pounds).[2] More of the comparison group teenagers (20.9%) than experimental group teenagers (16.5%) had low-birth-weight babies, but, once again, the group difference was not significant.

The 3-minute Apgar score in the two groups was quite similar— 7.3 for the experimental group and 6.7 for the comparison group. This small difference was nonsignificant.

Finally, the teenagers were compared with respect to their adoption of birth control 6 months after delivering their babies. For this

[2]All mothers gave birth to live infants; however, there were two neonatal deaths within 24 hours of birth in the comparison group.

variable, teenagers were coded as users of contraception if they were either using some method of birth control at the time of the follow-up interview or if they were nonusers but were sexually inactive (i.e., were using abstinence to prevent a repeat pregnancy). The results of the chi-squared test revealed that a significantly higher percentage of experimental group teenagers (81.7%) than comparison group teenagers (62.5%) reported using birth control after delivery. This difference was significant beyond the .01 level.

DISCUSSION

The results of this evaluation were disappointing, but not discouraging. There was only one outcome for which a significant difference was observed. The experimental program significantly increased the percentage of teenagers who used birth control after delivering their babies. Thus, one highly important result of participating in the program is that an early repeat pregnancy will be postponed. There is abundant research that has shown that repeat pregnancy among teenagers is especially damaging to their educational and occupational attainment and leads to particularly adverse labor and delivery outcomes in the higher-order births (Klugman, 1985; Jackson, 1978).

The experimental group had more prenatal care, but not significantly more. Perhaps part of the difficulty is that the program can only begin to deliver services once pregnancy has been diagnosed. If a teenager does not come in for a pregnancy test until her fourth or fifth month, this obviously puts an upper limit on the number of visits she will have; it also gives less time for her to eat properly, avoid smoking and drinking, and take other steps to enhance her health during pregnancy. Thus, one implication of this finding is that the program needs to do more to encourage early pregnancy screening. Perhaps a joint effort between the clinic personnel and school nurses in neighboring middle schools and high schools could be launched to publicize the need for a timely pregnancy test and to inform teenagers where such a test could be obtained. The two groups performed similarly with respect to the various labor and delivery outcomes chosen to evaluate the effectiveness of the new program. The issue of timeliness is again relevant here. The program may have been delivering services too late in the pregnancy for the instruction to have made much of an impact on the health of the mother and her child. This interpretation is supported, in part, by the fact that the one variable for which timeliness was *not* an issue (postpartum contraception) was, indeed, positively affected by program participation. Another possible implication is that the program itself should be made more powerful, for example, by lengthening or adding to instructional sessions.

Given that the experimental and comparison group differences were all in the hypothesized direction, it is also tempting to criticize the sample size. A larger sample (which was originally planned) might have yielded some significant differences.

In summary, the experimental intervention is not without promise. A particularly exciting finding is that participation in the program resulted in better contraceptive use, which will presumably lower the incidence of repeat pregnancy. It would be interesting to follow these teenagers two years after delivery to see if the groups differ in the rates of repeat pregnancy. It appears that more needs to be done to get these teenagers into the program early in their pregnancies. Perhaps then the true effectiveness of the program would be demonstrated.

CRITIQUE OF THE RESEARCH REPORT

In the following discussion, we present some comments on various aspects of this research report. You are urged to read the report and formulate your own opinion about its strengths and weaknesses before reading this critique. An evaluation of a study is necessarily partly subjective. Therefore, you might disagree with some of the points made below, and you might have additional criticisms and comments. We believe, however, that most of the serious methodologic flaws of the study are highlighted in our critique.

Title

The title for the study is misleading. The research does *not* investigate the role of health care professionals in serving the needs of pregnant teenagers. A more appropriate title would be "Health-Related Effects of an Intervention for Pregnant Teenagers."

Background

The background section of this report consists of three distinct elements that can be analyzed separately: a literature review, statement of the problem, and a theoretical framework.

The literature review is relatively clearly written and well organized. It serves the important function of establishing a need for the experimental program by documenting the prevalence of teenage pregnancy and some of its adverse consequences. However, the literature review could be improved. First, an inspection of the citations suggests that the author is not as up-to-date on research relating to teenage pregnancy as she might have been. Most of the references are from the early 1990s or even earlier, meaning that this literature review is about a decade old. Second, there is material in the literature review section that is not relevant and should be removed. For example, the paragraph on the options with which a pregnant teenager is faced (paragraph 3) is not germane to the research problem. A third and more critical flaw is what the review does *not* cover. Given the research problem, there are probably four main points that should be addressed in the review:

1. How widespread is teenage pregnancy and parenthood?
2. What are the social and health consequences of early child-bearing?
3. What has been done (especially by nurses) to address the problems associated with teenage parenthood?
4. How successful have other interventions been?

The review adequately handles the first question: The need for concern is established. The second question is covered in the review, but perhaps more depth and more recent research is needed here. The new study is based on an assumption of negative health outcomes in teenaged mothers. The author has strung together a series of references without giving the reader any clues about the reliability of the information. The author would have made her point more convincingly if she had added a sentence such as "For example, in a carefully executed prospective study involving nearly 8000 pregnant women, Beach (1987) found that young maternal age was significantly associated with higher rates of prematurity and other negative neonatal outcomes." The third and fourth points that should have been covered are totally absent from the review. Surely the author's experimental program does not represent the first attempt to address the needs of pregnant teenagers. How is Nelson's intervention different from or better than other interventions? What reason does she have to believe that such an intervention might be successful? Nelson has provided a rationale for addressing the problem but no rationale for the manner in which she has addressed it. If, in fact, there is little information about other interventions and their effectiveness in improving health outcomes, then the review should say so.

The problem statement and hypothesis were stated succinctly and clearly. The hypothesis is complex (there are multiple dependent variables) and directional (it predicts better outcomes among teenagers participating in the special program).

The third component of the background section of the report is the theoretical framework. In our opinion, the theoretical framework chosen does little to enhance the research. The hypothesis is not generated on the basis of the model, nor does the intervention itself grow out of the model. One gets the feeling that the model was slapped on as an afterthought to try to make the study seem more sophisticated or theoretical. Actually, if more thought had been given to this conceptual framework, it might have proved useful. According to this model, the most immediate and direct influences on a pregnant teenager are her family, friends, and sexual partner. One programmatic implication of this is that the intervention should involve one or more of these influences. For example, a workshop for the teenagers' parents could have been developed to reinforce the teenagers' need for adequate nutrition and prenatal care. A research hypothesis that could have been tested in the context of the model is that teenagers who are missing one of the direct influences would be especially susceptible to the influence of less proximal health care providers (i.e., the program). For example, it might be hypothesized that pregnant teenagers who do not live with both parents have to depend on alternative sources of social support (such as health care personnel) during the pregnancy. Thus, it is not that the theoretical context selected is far-fetched but rather that it was not convincingly linked to the actual research problem. Perhaps an alternative theoretical context would have been better. Or perhaps the researcher simply should have been honest and admitted that her research was practical, not theoretical.

Methods

The design used to test the research hypothesis was a widely used preexperimental design. Two groups, whose equivalence is assumed but not established, were compared on several outcome measures. The design is one that has serious problems because the preintervention comparability of the groups is unknown.

The most serious threat to the internal validity of the study is selection bias. Selection bias can work both ways to mask true treatment effects or to create the illusion of a program effect when none exists. This is because selection bias can be either positive (i.e., the experimental group can be initially advantaged in relation to the comparison group) or negative (i.e., the experimental group can have pretreatment disadvantages). In the present study, it is possible that the two hospitals served clients of different economic circumstances, for example. If the average income of the families of the experimental group teenagers was higher, then these teenagers would probably have a better opportunity for adequate prenatal nutrition than the comparison group teenagers. Or the comparison hospital might serve older teens, a higher percentage of married teens, or a higher percentage of teens attending a special school-based program for pregnant students. None of these extraneous variables, which could affect the mother's health, has been controlled.

Another way in which the design was vulnerable to selection bias is the high refusal rate in the experimental group. Of the 217 eligible teenagers, half declined to participate in the special program. We cannot assume that the 109 girls who participated were a random sample of the eligible girls. Again, biases could be either positive or negative. A positive selection bias would be created if, for example, the teenagers who were the most motivated to have a healthy pregnancy selected themselves into the experimental group. A negative selection bias would result if the teenagers from the most disadvantaged households or from families offering little support elected to participate in the program. In the comparison group, hospital records were used primarily to collect the data, so this self-selection problem could not occur (except for refusals to answer the contraceptive questions six months postpartum).

The researcher could have taken a number of steps to either control selection biases or, at the least, estimate their direction and magnitude. The following are among the most critical extraneous variables: social class and family income, age, race and ethnicity, parity, participation in another pregnant teenager program, marital status, and prepregnancy experience with contraception (for the postpartum contraception outcome). The researcher should have attempted to gather information on these variables from experimental group and comparison group teenagers *and* from eligible teenagers in the experimental hospital who declined to participate in the program. To the extent that these three groups were found to be similar on these variables, credibility in the internal validity of the study would be enhanced. If sizable differences were observed, the researcher would at least know or suspect the direction of the biases and could factor that information into her interpretation and conclusions.

Had the researcher gathered information on the extraneous variables, another possibility would have been to match experimental and comparison group subjects on one or two variables, such as family income and age. Matching is not an ideal method of controlling extraneous variables; for one thing, matching on two variables would not equate the two groups in terms of the other extraneous variables. However, matching is preferable to doing nothing to control extraneous variation.

So far we have focused our attention on the research design, but other aspects of the study are also problematic. Let us consider the decision the researcher made about the population. The target population is not explicitly defined by the researcher, but one can infer that the target population is pregnant young women under age 20 who carry their infants to delivery. The accessible population is pregnant teenagers from one area in Chicago. Is it reasonable to assume that the accessible population is representative of the target population? No, it is not. It is likely that the accessible population is quite different with regard to health care, family intactness, and many other characteristics. The researcher should have more clearly discussed exactly who was the target population of this research.

Nelson would have done well, in fact, to delimit the target population; had she done so, it might have been possible to control some of the extraneous variables discussed previously. For example, Nelson could have established eligibility criteria that excluded multigravidas, very young teenagers (e.g., under age 15), or married teenagers. Such a specification would have limited the generalizability of the findings, but it would have enhanced the internal validity of the study because it probably would have increased the comparability of the experimental and comparison groups.

The sample was a sample of convenience, the least effective sampling design for a quantitative study. There is no way of knowing whether the sample represents the accessible and target populations. Although probability sampling likely was not feasible, the researcher might have improved her sampling design by using a quota sampling plan. For example, if the researcher knew that in the accessible population, half of the families received public assistance, then it might have been possible to enhance the representativeness of the samples by using a quota system to ensure that half of the research subjects came from welfare-dependent families.

Sample size is a difficult issue. Many of the reported results were in the hypothesized direction but were nonsignificant. When this is the case, the adequacy of the sample size is always suspect, as Nelson pointed out. Each group had about 100 subjects. In many cases, this sample size would be considered adequate, but in the present case, it is not. One of the difficulties in testing the effectiveness of new interventions is that, generally, the experimental group is not being compared with a no-treatment group. Although the comparison group in this example was not getting the special program services, it cannot be assumed that this group was getting no services at all. Some comparison group members may have had ample prenatal care during which the health care staff may have provided much of the same information as they taught in the special program. The point is not that the new program was not needed but rather that unless an intervention is extremely powerful and innovative, the incremental improvement will typically be rather small. When relatively small effects are anticipated, the sample must be very large for differences to be statistically significant. Although it is beyond the scope of this book to explain the power analysis calculations, it can be shown that to detect a significant difference between the two groups with respect, say, to the incidence of toxemia, a sample of over 5000 pregnant teenagers would have been needed. Had the researcher done a power analysis before conducting the study, she might have realized the insufficiency of her sample for some of the outcomes and might have developed a different sampling plan or identified different dependent variables.

The third major methodologic decision concerns the measurement of the research variables. For the most part, the researcher did a good job in selecting objective, reliable, and valid outcome measures. Also, her operational definitions were clearly worded and unambiguous. Two comments are in order, however. First, it might have been better to operationalize two of the variables differently. Infant birth weight might have been more sensitively measured as actual weight (a ratio-level measurement) or as a three-level ordinal variable (< 1500 grams; > 1500 but < 2500 grams; and > 2500 grams) instead of as a dichotomous variable. The contraceptive variable could also have been operationalized to yield a more sensitive (i.e., more discriminating) measure. Rather than measuring contraceptive use as a dichotomy, Nelson could have created an ordinal scale based on either frequency of use (e.g., 0%, 1% to 25%, 26% to 50%, 51% to 75%, and 76% to 100% of the time) or on the effectiveness of the *type* of birth control used.

A second consideration is whether the outcome variables adequately captured the effects of program activities. It might have been easier, with the small sample of 229 teenagers, and more directly relevant to capture group differences in, say, dietary practices during pregnancy than in infant birth weight. None of the outcome variables measured the effects of parenting education. In other words, the researcher could have added more direct measures of the effects of the special program.

One other point about the methods should be made, and that relates to ethical considerations. The article does not specifically say that subjects were asked for their informed consent, but that does not necessarily mean that no written consent was obtained. It is quite likely that the experimental group subjects, when asked to volunteer for the special program, were advised about their participation in the study and asked to sign a consent form. But what about the control group subjects? The article implies that comparison group members were given no opportunity to decline participation and were not aware of having their birth outcomes used as data in the research. In some cases, this procedure is acceptable. For example, a hospital or clinic might agree to release patient information without the patients' consent if the release of such information is done anonymously—that is, if it can be provided in such a way that even the researcher does not know the identity of the patients. In the present study, however, it is clear that the names of the comparison subjects *were* given to the researcher since she had to contact the comparison group at six months postpartum to determine their contraceptive practices. Thus, this study does not appear to have adequately safeguarded the rights of the comparison group subjects.

In summary, the researcher appears not to have adhered to ethical procedures, and she also failed to give the new program a fair test. Nelson should have taken a number of steps to control extraneous variables and should have attempted to get a larger sample (even if this meant waiting for additional subjects to enroll in the program). In addition to concerns about the internal validity of the study, its generalizability is also questionable.

Results

Nelson did a good job of presenting the results of the study. The presentation was straightforward and succinct and was enhanced by the inclusion of a good table and figures. The style of this section was also appropriate: It was written objectively and was well organized.

The statistical analyses were also reasonably well done. The descriptive statistics (means and percentages) were appropriate for the level of measurement of the variables. The author did not, however, provide any information about the variability of the measures, except for noting the range for the "time spent in labor" variable. Figure 15-B suggests that the two groups did differ in variability: The comparison group was more heterogeneous than the experimental group with regard to prenatal care received.

The two types of inferential statistics used (the t-test and chi-squared test) were also appropriate, given the levels of measurement of the outcome variables. The results of these tests were efficiently presented in a single table. It should be noted that there are more powerful statistics available that could have been used to control extraneous variables (e.g., analysis of covariance), but in the present study, it appears that the only extraneous variable that could have been controlled through statistical procedures was the subjects' ages because no data were apparently collected on other extraneous variables (social class, ethnicity, parity, and so on).

Discussion

Nelson's discussion section fails almost entirely to take the study's limitations into account in interpreting the data. The one exception is her acknowledgment that the sample size was too small. She seems unconcerned about the many threats to the internal or external validity of her research.

Nelson lays almost all the blame for the nonsignificant findings on the program rather than on the research methods. She feels that two aspects of the program should be changed: (1) recruitment of teenagers into the program earlier in their pregnancies and (2) strengthening program services. Both recommendations might be worth pursuing, but there is little in the data to suggest these modifications. With nonsignificant results such as those that predominated in this study, there are two possibilities to consider: (1) the results are accurate—that is, the program is not effective for those outcomes examined (though it might be effective for other measures), and (2) the results are false—that is, the existing program is effective for the outcomes examined, but the tests failed to demonstrate it. Nelson concluded that the first possibility was correct and therefore recommended that the program be changed. Equally plausible is the possibility that the study methods were too weak to demonstrate the program's true effects.

We do not have enough information about the characteristics of the sample to conclude with certainty that there were substantial selection biases. We do, however, have a clue that selection biases were operative in a direction that would make the program look less effective than it actually is. Nelson noted in the beginning of the results section that the average age of the teenagers in the experimental group was 17.1, compared with 18.0 in the comparison group. Age is inversely related to positive labor and delivery outcomes, indeed, that is the basis for having a special program for teenaged mothers. Therefore, the experimental group's performance on the outcome measures was possibly depressed by the youth of that group. Had the two groups been equivalent in terms of age, the group differences might have been larger and could have reached levels of statistical significance. Other uncontrolled pretreatment differences could also have masked true treatment effects.

For the one significant outcome, we cannot rule out the possibility that a Type I error was made—that is, that the null hypothesis was in fact true. Again, selection biases could have been operative. The experimental group might have contained many more girls who had preprogram experience with contraception; it might have contained more highly motivated teenagers, or more single teenagers, or more teenagers who had already had multiple pregnancies than the comparison group. There simply is no way of knowing whether the significant outcome reflects true program effects or merely initial group differences.

Aside from Nelson's disregard for the problems of internal validity, the author definitely overstepped the bounds of scholarly speculation by reading too much into her data. She unquestionably assumed that the program *caused* contraceptive improvements: "the experimental program significantly increased the percentage of teenagers who used birth control. . . ." Worse yet, she went on to conclude that repeat pregnancies will be postponed in the experimental group, although she does not know whether the teenagers used an effective contraception, whether they used it all the time, or whether they used it correctly.

As another example of going beyond the data, Nelson became overly invested in her notion that teenagers need greater and earlier exposure to the program. It is not that her hypothesis has no merit—the problem is that she builds an elaborate rationale for program changes with no apparent empirical support. She probably had information on when in the pregnancy the teenagers entered the program, but that information was not shared with readers. Her argument about the need for more publicity on early screening would have had more clout if she had reported that most teenagers entered the program during the fourth month of their pregnancies or later. Additionally, she could have marshaled more evidence in support of her proposal if she had been able to show that earlier entry into the program was associated with better health outcomes. For example, she could have compared the outcomes of teenagers entering the program in the first, second, and third trimesters of their pregnancies.

In conclusion, the study has several positive features. As Nelson noted, there is some reason to be cautiously optimistic that the program *could* have some beneficial effects. However, the existing study is too seriously flawed to reach any conclusions, even tentatively. A replication with improved research methods clearly is needed to solve the research problem.

2. At the end of this Study Guide, in Part VII, are two actual research reports, one for a quantitative study and the other for a qualitative study. Read one or both of these reports and prepare a three- to five-page critique summarizing the major strengths and weaknesses of the study.

■ E. Special Projects

1. Rewrite Nelson's report (Exercise D.1), using some of the suggestions from the critique or from classroom discussions.

2. Prepare a list of ten critical questions that would need to be addressed in a critique of the methodological dimensions of a quantitative study. Select a recent research report for a quantitative study and apply those questions to it.

3. Prepare a list of ten critical questions that would need to be addressed in a critique of the methodological dimensions of a qualitative study. Select a recent research report for a qualitative study and apply those questions to it.

CHAPTER 16

Using Research Findings in Nursing Practice

■ A. Matching Exercises

1. Match each of the strategies from Set B with one (or more) of the roles indicated in Set A. Indicate the letter corresponding to your response next to each of the strategies in Set B.

SET A

a. Nursing researchers
b. Nursing faculty and educators
c. Practicing nurses and nursing students
d. Nursing administrators

SET B   **RESPONSES**

1. Become involved in a journal club.   _____

2. Perform replications.   _____

3. Prepare integrative reviews of research literature.   _____

4. Offer resources for utilization projects.   _____

5. Disseminate findings.   _____

6. Specify clinical implications of findings.   _____

7. Read research reports critically.   _____

8. Foster intellectual curiosity in the work environment.   _____

9. Provide a forum for communication between clinicians
   and researchers.   _____

10. Expect evidence that a procedure is effective.   _____

■ B. Completion Exercises

Write the words or phrases that correctly complete the sentences below.

1. _____ refers to the use of some aspect of a scientific investigation in an application unrelated to the original research.

2. There is considerable concern about the _____ between knowledge production and knowledge utilization.

3. The most well-known nursing research utilization project, conducted in Michigan, is the _____ Project.

4. For research results to be believable and trustworthy, study findings must be _____ in several different settings.

5. The _____ model of utilization provides guidance for an individual utilization effort.

6. In the Iowa Model of Research in Practice, the two starting points for an organizational utilization project are referred to as _____ trigger and _____ trigger.

7. The three broad classes of criteria for research utilization are clinical relevance, scientific merit, and _____.

8. The issue of _____ concerns whether it makes sense to implement an innovation in a new practice setting.

9. A cost/benefit assessment should consider not only the net cost or gain of implementing an innovation but also _____.

10. A utilization project should include a(n) _____ component to determine the effectiveness of the innovation.

■ C. Study Questions

1. Define the following terms. Compare your definition with the definition in Chapter 16 of the textbook or in the Glossary.

   a. Instrumental utilization _____

   _____

   b. Conceptual utilization _____

   _____

c. Knowledge creep _____

_____

d. Decision accretion _____

_____

e. Awareness stage of adoption _____

_____

f. Persuasion state of adoption _____

_____

g. Scientific merit _____

_____

h. Cost/benefit ratio _____

_____

i. Problem-focused trigger _____

_____

j. Knowledge-focused trigger _____

_____

k. Research-based nursing protocol _____

_____

2. Prepare an example of a research question that could be posed to improve nursing care in the five phases of the nursing process.

a. Assessment phase _____

_____

b. Diagnosis phase _____

_____

c. Planning phase _____

_____

d. Intervention phase _____

_____

e. Evaluation phase _____

_____

3. Think about a nursing procedure about which you have been instructed. Determine whether the procedure is based on scientific evidence indicating that the procedure is effective. If it is not based on scientific evidence, on what is it based, and why do you think scientific evidence was not used?

_____

_____

_____

_____

_____

4. Identify the factors in your own setting that you think facilitate or inhibit research utilization (or, in an educational setting, the factors that promote or inhibit a climate in which research utilization is valued).

_____

_____

_____

_____

_____

5. Read either Brett's (1987) article regarding the adoption of fourteen nursing innovations ("Use of nursing practice research findings," *Nursing Research, 36,* 344–349) or the more recent (1990) replication study based on the same fourteen innovations by Coyle and Sokop ("Innovation adoption behavior among nurses," *Nursing Research, 39,* 176–180). For each of the fourteen innovations, indicate whether you yourself are aware of the findings, persuaded that the findings should be used, use the findings sometimes in a clinical situation, or use the findings always in a clinical situation.

1. _____

_____

2. _____

_____

3. _____

_____

4. _____

_____

5. _____

6. _____

7. _____

8. _____

9. _____

10. _____

11. _____

12. _____

13. _____

14. _____

6. With regard to the fourteen innovations selected in Brett's study (see Exercise 5 above), select an innovation or finding of which you (or most class members) were unaware. Go to the original source and read the research report. Perform a critique of the study, indicating in particular why you think there may have been barriers to having the innovation implemented in a local setting.

_____

_____

_____

_____

■ D. Application Exercise

1. Below are several suggested research articles. Read one or more of these articles, paying special attention to the Conclusions/Implications section of the report. Evaluate the extent to which you believe the researchers' discussion would facilitate the utilization of the study findings within clinical settings. If possible, suggest some clinical implications that the researchers did not discuss.

   ■ Baldwin, I. C., & Heland, M. (2000). Incidence of cardiac dysrhythmias in patients during pulmonary artery catheter removal after cardiac surgery. *Heart & Lung, 29,* 155–160.

   ■ Cioffi, J. (2000). Recognition of patients who require emergency assistance. *Heart & Lung, 29,* 262–268.

   ■ Corrarino, J. E., Williams, C., Campbell, W. S., Amrhein, E., LoPiano, L., & Kalachik, D. (2000). Linking substance-abusing pregnant women to drug treatment services: A pilot program. *Journal of Obstetric, Gynecologic, and Neonatal Nursing, 29,* 369–376.

   ■ Fuller, B. F. (2000). Fluctuations in established infant pain behaviors. *Clinical Nursing Research, 9,* 298–316.

   ■ Hansebo, G., & Kihlgren, M. (2000). Patient life stories and current situation as told by carers in nursing home wards. *Clinical Nursing Research, 9,* 260–279.

   ■ Jacobs, V. (2000). Informational needs of surgical patients following discharge. *Applied Nursing Research, 13,* 12–18.

   ■ Keller, M. L., vonSadovszky, V., Pankratz, B., & Hermsen, J. (2000). Self-disclosure of HPV infection to sexual partners. *Western Journal of Nursing Research, 22,* 285–302.

   ■ Li, H., Stewart, B. J., Imle, M. A., Archbold, P. G., & Felver, L. (2000). Families and hospitalized elders: A typology of family care actions. *Research in Nursing and Health, 23,* 3–16.

■ E. Special Project

1. Select a study from the nursing research literature. Using the utilization criteria indicated in Box 16-2 of the textbook, assess the potential for utilizing the study results in a clinical practice setting. If the study meets the three major classes of criteria for utilization, develop a utilization plan.

2. The textbook described a utilization project conducted under the auspices of the Association of Women's Health, Obstetric, and Neonatal Nurses (AWHONN) that focused on urinary incontinence for women. The following articles describe an earlier AWHONN utilization project:

■ Meier, P. P. (1994). Transition of the preterm infant to an open crib: Process of the project group. *Journal of Obstetric, Gynecologic, and Neonatal Nursing, 23*, 321–326.

■ Medoff-Cooper, B. (1994). Transition of the preterm infant to an open crib. *Journal of Obstetric, Gynecologic, and Neonatal Nursing, 23*, 329–335.

■ Gelhar, D. K., Miserendino, C. A., O'Sullivan, P. L., & Vessey, J. A. (1994). Research from the research utilization project: Environmental temperatures. *Journal of Obstetric, Gynecologic, and Neonatal Nursing, 23*, 341–344.

Read these reports and evaluate the efficacy of this utilization project.

PART VII

Research Reports

Patient Outcomes for the Chronically Critically Ill: Special Care Unit Versus Intensive Care Unit

Ellen B. Rudy, Barbara J. Daly,
Sara Douglas, Hugo D. Montenegro,
Rhayun Song, Mary Ann Dyer

The purpose of this study was to compare the effects of a low-technology environment of care and a nurse case management case delivery system (special care unit, SCU) with the traditional high-technology environment (ICU) and primary nursing care delivery system on the patient outcomes of length of stay, mortality, readmission, complications, satisfaction, and cost. A sample of 220 chronically critically ill patients were randomly assigned to either the SCU (n = 145) or the ICU (n = 75). Few significant differences were found between the two groups in length of stay, mortality, or complications. However, the findings showed significant cost savings in the SCU group in the charges accrued during the study period and in the charges and costs to produce a survivor. The average total cost of delivering care was $5,000 less per patient in the SCU than in the traditional ICU. In addition, the cost to produce a survivor was $19,000 less in the SCU. Results from this 4-year clinical trial demonstrate that nurse case managers in a SCU setting can produce patient outcomes equal to or better than those in the traditional ICU care environment for long-term critically ill patients.

The original purpose of intensive care units (ICUs) was to locate groups of patients together who had similar needs for specialized monitoring and care so that highly trained health care personnel would be available to meet these specialized needs. As the success of ICUs has grown and expanded, the as-

Published in *Nursing Research* (1995), 44, 324–331.

sumption that a typical ICU patient will require only a short length of stay in the unit during the most acute phase of an illness has given way to the recognition that stays of more than 1 month are not uncommon (Berenson, 1984; Daly, Rudy, Thompson, & Happ, 1991).

These long-stay ICU patients represent a challenge to the current system, not only because of costs, but also because of concern for patient outcomes. These patients are often elderly, have underlying chronic conditions that complicate or exacerbate their acute illness, and often require sustained ventilatory and nutritional support. A prime example of these types of patients are those referred to as "ventilator dependent," found to varying degrees in nearly every ICU in the country (American Association for Respiratory Care, 1991).

The term "chronically critically ill" has been previously used (Daly et al., 1991) to describe patients who have extended stays in the ICU. These patients have become the most burdensome to nurses and physicians, who see their progress as slow and frustrating, to hospital administrators because of the extended bed occupancy in times of high demand, and to hospital financial officers because of costs that usually exceed the diagnosis-related group (DRG) cost allocation. Patients who have ICU length of stays greater than 21 days account for approximately 3% of the total number of patients admitted to the ICUs, yet they account for approximately 25% to 38% of the patient days (Daly et al., 1991).

While ample evidence confirms that this subpopulation of ICU patients represents a drain on hospital resources, few studies have attempted to evaluate the effects of a care delivery system outside the ICU setting on patient outcomes, costs, and nurse outcomes. The majority of studies that have examined ICU patient outcomes have been limited primarily to mortality and length of stay (Bersenson, 1984; Borlase, Baxter, Benotti, Stone, et al., 1991; Madoff, Sharpe, Fath, Simons, & Cerra, 1985). More recently, attention has been given to cost in terms of risk-adjusted ICU length of stays, cost and utility of diagnostic and laboratory tests, and time on mechanical ventilation (Gundlach & Faulkner, 1991; Kappstein, Schulgen, Beyer, Geiger, et al., 1992; Roberts Bell, Ostryzniuk, Dobson, et al., 1993; Schapira, Studnicki, Bradham, Wolff, & Jarrett, 1993; Zimmerman, Shortell, Knaus, Rousseau, et al., 1993).

In studies limited to mechanically ventilated patients, comparisons on length of stay and costs have been examined in "a before-and-after" design following initiation of a ventilatory management team (Cohen, Bari, Strosbug, Weinberg, et al., 1991), on overall costs for mechanically ventilated patients cared for in an ICU versus a noninvasive respiratory care unit (Elpern, Silver, Rosen, & Bone, 1991), and on hospital charges and life expectancy for elderly mechanically ventilated ICU patients (Cohen, Lambrinos, & Fein, 1993). The lack of randomized trials comparing care delivery systems for these high-cost patients is noteworthy, as well as the limitation of outcome measurements to mortality and cost.

The purpose of the current study was to compare the effects of a low-technology environment of care based on a nurse-managed care delivery system [special care unit (SCU) environment] with the traditional high-technology ICU environment based on a primary nursing care delivery system. The two groups were compared on the outcomes of length of stay, mortality, readmission to the hospital, complications, patient and family satisfaction, and cost. The complications were defined as number and type of infections, number and type of respiratory complications, and number and type of life-threatening complications.

■ Method

Sample: A total of 276 subjects were eligible for the study. Table 1 lists eligibility criteria. Only four refused to participate; of the remaining 272 subjects, 220 (81%) were able to be randomized. Of the 52 subjects who were not randomly assigned to a treatment group, the majority (n = 37, 71%) were due to bed availability, with only 13 (25%) due to physician refusal to allow randomization to treatment assignment, and 2 (4%) because of family unwillingness to allow treatment assignment.

The final sample for analysis consisted of 145 subjects cared for in the SCU environment and 75 subjects in the ICU environment. The sample was nearly equally divided between males and females, was predominantly white (70%), with an average age of 64 years (range 16 to 90 years). The groups were equivalent on gender, age, and race, on the prior ICU length of stay (M = 16 days, SD = 13.3), and on the general medical diagnosis of patients. Significant differences were found in the type of ICU where patients received

Table 1.   Eligibility Criteria for Patients in the Study

Length of stay (LOS) in ICU >5 days[a]

Not currently receiving IV vasopressor (exception: low-level maintenance drip)

No pulmonary artery monitor required

No acute event (arrest, unstable event) in past 3 days

APACHE II 18 or less

TISS class II or III (10 to 39 points)

Unable to be cared for on a general nursing unit

NOTE. APACHE, Acute physiological and chronic health evaluation; TISS, Therapeutic intervention scoring system.

[a]First 2 years of study LOS in ICU was >7 days, but with experience the LOS was shortened to ≥5 days.

their care prior to the study and in source of payment for care. A higher percentage of no payment source and private insurance was found in the ICU group, with a higher percentage of public (Medicare and Medicaid) insurance in the SCU group.

To ensure similarity in acuity of illness between the two groups of subjects, a variety of variables were compared. No significant difference between the groups was noted on the Acute Physiological and Chronic Health Evaluation II (APACHE II) on admission to the ICU or at time of eligibility for the study, the Therapeutic Intervention Scoring System (TISS) at the time of eligibility for the study, and the number of infections prior to admission to the study. In terms of these known risk predictors, then, the experimental and control groups were equivalent. There were, however significantly ($p \le .03$) more respiratory complications prior to the study in the patients admitted to the SCU. While statistically significant, in practical terms, the means of the two groups varied by only 0.5, with a very similar range and standard deviation. Furthermore, the higher risk from prior respiratory complications was in the SCU sample, so claims that patients in the ICU were sicker can be refuted.

Setting: The environments of care were conceptualized according to the sociotechnical theory of work, which proposes that both the physical environment in which work occurs, the procedures and processes of work, and the way workers interact with one another and with the environment will influence the way in which the work is accomplished and ultimately the output of the work (Happ, 1993; Pasmore, 1988, Pasmore & Sherwood, 1978).

The SCU environment of care was designed to decrease technology and ensure privacy in order to promote sleep and rest, allow for more freedom for interaction with family and friends, ensure continuity of care by nurse case managers working with medical protocols, and create an opportunity for a self-directed governance model. The significant contrasting features of the SCU versus the ICU were the physical environment, the nursing practice model, and the nursing management model.

The SCU environment was a 7-bed unit with only private rooms. Technology was limited to electrocardiographic monitors, ventilators, and occasional arterial pressure monitoring. Family involvement was encouraged through unlimited visiting and overnight accommodations. The care delivery system was case management, with the nurse case manager accountable clinically and financially for each patient's outcomes. Interns and residents were not in the unit. Each patient's plan of care was established, coordinated, and evaluated by the case manager working in close collaboration with the unit's attending physician. Case managers participated in an 8-week training program for the SCU and, with the medical director of the unit, developed protocols that addressed such activities as ventilator weaning, nutrition, pain management, and sedation. In addition, the SCU initiated a shared governance management model, which vested the authority and responsibility for managing the work environment in the staff nurses.

The ICU environments included primarily a 12-bed medical intensive care unit and an 18-bed surgical intensive care unit. A small percentage of subjects

(19%) who met the study criteria came from the neurosurgical intensive care unit or the coronary intensive care unit. The majority (80%) of bed spaces were open or curtained off from a central nursing station. Visitor lounges were outside the units, family visiting was controlled, and overnight stays were not accommodated. Technology and physiological monitoring devices were not limited, and lighting and noise from the overall unit was difficult to exclude from the patient bed spaces. A primary nursing model of care was used in all of the ICUs, with total nursing care the responsibility of the primary nurse. Interns and residents delivered most of the medical care, as is the standard practice in academic medical centers. A bureaucratic management model was used with centralized decision making at the head nurse level, and organizational responsibility and authority descending within each unit through a distinct chain of command.

Procedure: Rounds were made every other day in all ICUs to assess patient eligibility. Using a coin toss, eligible patients were assigned to either the experimental or control group. Consent to participate was then obtained from both the primary physician and the patient. If the patient was unable to consent, the next of kin was asked for permission. If the patients and their physicians consented, patients were then enrolled and, if in the experimental group, transferred to the SCU. This procedure for consent and group assignment was approved by the hospital's Institutional Review Board.

Every effort was made to randomize subject assignment to groups, but because of the practical need to keep the 7-bed SCU occupied, a distribution of approximately 2:1 was needed to meet this obligation. Based on various options for randomization of subject assignment in the clinical trials literature (Efron, 1971; Hjelm-Karlsson, 1991; Meinert & Tonasicia, 1986), a biased-coin format was used in which two out of every three eligible subjects were assigned to the experimental group (SCU), and one was assigned to the control (Rudy, Vaska, Daly, Happ, & Shiao, 1993). While this design helped to ensure a more steady occupancy of the SCU, the disadvantage was that at certain times the investigator knew ahead of time where the next eligible patient would be assigned. Efforts were made to overcome this bias. First, the date on which a patient became eligible for the study was used to determine who was next in line for assignment, and this was outside the direct control of the investigators. Second, caregivers in both the SCU and ICU were not involved in determining patient eligibility or patient assignments. Furthermore, patients transferred to SCU because of a low census in the SCU rather than through the randomized assignment were not part of the study sample. Even with these disadvantages, this assignment procedure was far superior to a simple comparative design without a randomization procedure, allowing real comparisons to occur within the limitations of a clinical setting.

Following group assignment and transfer of experimental subjects to the SCU, data collection was done prospectively. Patient records were reviewed at least every other day until the patient was discharged from the hospital or died.

Instruments: The ACUTE PHYSIOLOGICAL AND CHRONIC HEALTH EVALUATION II (APACHE II) was used to establish the similarity of severity of illness between the experimental and control groups and as a measure of severity of illness at entry to the study. This instrument, a refinement of the original APACHE (Knaus, Draper, Wagner, & Zimmerman, 1986), is a severity of disease classification system that predicts risk of death. It is based on the assumption that the severity of disease can be quantified by the degree of abnormality of physiologic variables in combination with age and the presence of chronic disease. The range of possible scores is 0 to 71. Accuracy in predicting death was found to be 86% in a study of 5,815 patients (Knaus et al., 1986). This is consistent with earlier studies in which regression analysis was used to validate mortality prediction using the acute physiology portion of the tool (Wagner, Knaus, & Draper, 1983). In a multihospital study of critically ill patients that used the APACHE classification, an interrater agreement of .95 was maintained (Knaus et al., 1986).

The THERAPEUTIC INTERVENTION SCORING SYSTEM (TISS) (Keene & Cullen, 1983) was designed to classify intensive care patients according to intensity of resource utilization. The TISS score is obtained by recording the number of weighted interventions actually used on the patient from a list of 76. The range of total scores is 0 to 181. TISS has been used since 1974 in multiple studies to assess severity of illness, outcomes of critical care, and utilization of ICU beds (Byrick, Mindorff, McKee, & Mudge, 1980; Schwartz & Cullen, 1981), and recently to examine the relationship between charges and reimbursement in different patient populations (Bekes, Fleming, & Scott, 1988; Teres, Rapaport, Lemeshow, Haber, et al., 1988). It was used in this study to compare utilization of resources in groups matched for severity of illness by APACHE. Validity is based on the initial study by Cullen, Civetta, Briggs, and Ferrara (1974) who recorded all interventions according to critically ill subjects and subsequently divided these into classes to be used to describe resource utilization: Class I = 0 to 9, Class II = 10 to 19, Class III = 20 to 39, Class IV ≥ 40. Experts in critical care validated the list of interventions as adequately and accurately reflecting critical care patient management (Byrick et al., 1980; Schwartz & Cullen, 1981). Four experienced ICU nurses were trained in the use of TISS and 20 critically ill patients were evaluated at the start of this study, each by two nurses within 1 hour of each other. The correlation coefficient for this interrater reliability was $r = .96$.

The LAMONICA-OBERST PATIENT SATISFACTION SCALE measures satisfaction with care, defined as the degree of congruence between patients' expectations of nursing care and their perceptions of care actually received (LaMonica, Oberst, Madea, & Wolf, 1986). Three dimensions of nursing care are measured: technical-professional, trusting relationship, and education relationship. The scale was based on the Risser scale (1975) and was modified to be appropriate for the acute care setting. Internal consistency of the three subscales in separate studies ranged from .80 to .90. The LaMonica-Oberst instrument consisted of 41 statements about nursing care to which the patient indicated agreement or disagreement using a Likert scale.

After preliminary use in this study, it became apparent that the instrument was too difficult for patients who were recovering from a critical illness to complete. Following a factor analysis, the scale was shortened to 15 items by removing items that demonstrated redundancy. Post-hoc analysis identified three factors. The alpha coefficient for the revised Patient Satisfaction scale has averaged .92 ($n = 93$). Construct validity is supported in that the identified factors are the same as those identified in LaMonica's original work.

A similar analysis was performed on the Family Satisfaction scale. This instrument was developed from the LaMonica-Oberst Patient Satisfaction scale by changing the wording of items to reflect the family member's satisfaction with the care received by the patient. This scale was shortened from the original 41 items to 29 items.

The RESPIRATORY COMPLICATIONS INDEX (RCI) was developed by the investigators. It is a checklist that is easily administered and scored. It includes the categories of respiratory complications evident in critical care areas. The range of total possible scores is 0 to 10. The criteria used to determine the presence of a pulmonary complication include: radiologic reports of atelectasis, consolidation, or collapse; fever; arterial blood gas results; positive sputum cultures, and clinical signs as documented in progress notes. While this checklist was constructed specifically for the study, these criteria are routinely used by other investigators in studying frequency of pulmonary complications (Ali, Serrett, Wood, & Anthomisen, 1985; Kirilloff, Owens, Rogers, & Mazzocco, 1985; Morran, Finlay, Mathieson, McKay, et al., 1983). Some association between occurrences of individual complications can be expected. For example, respiratory infections may commonly be associated with increased likelihood of hypoxia or failure to wean. The construct validity of the instrument is supported by the data obtained from both preliminary studies and the special care unit. Rules for use of the tool were established in these preliminary studies and average interrater reliability of .94 was maintained.

The INFECTION COMPLICATIONS INDEX (ICI) is an investigator-developed checklist. It includes the specific sites of infections commonly found in critical care areas, as well as general indicators of infection. The checklist identifies critical indicators from the respiratory and urinary tracks, blood, and wound, as well as general indicators of present infections. The general criteria are considered to be positive critical indicators of infection of unknown source only when other noninfectious causes are absent. While this checklist was constructed specifically for the study, these criteria are routinely used by other investigators studying nosocomial infections (Bartlett, O'Keefe, Tally, Louie, & Gorbach, 1986; Garner & Favero, 1986; Parkhurst, Blaser, Laxson, & Wang, 1985).

Construct validity was established by testing the relationship between the total number of infections and length of hospital stay ($r = .78$) and ICU length of stay ($r = .88$). Interrater reliability was maintained at $\leq 90\%$ throughout the study.

The LIFE-THREATENING COMPLICATION INDEX (LTCI) was developed in the second year of the study when it became evident that the occurrence of such complications as seizures, ventricular fibrillation, and gastrointestinal bleeding were frequent enough that the rate of occurrence could serve as additional outcome measures. The LTCI includes 15 life-threatening events or episodes. To be counted as life threatening, the event must have required medical treatment.

The LTCI is scored by giving one point for each event. Scores range from 0 to 15. Construct validity is supported by the positive correlation between the LTCI and hospital mortality ($r = .24$), hospital length of stay ($r = .32$), and critical care days ($r = .40$). The interrater reliability averaged .97 over the four years of the study. Data for the LTCI were obtained retrospectively for those patients who had entered the study prior to the design of the instrument; for all other patients, the data were collected prospectively with the other outcome measures.

Since each instrument is dependent on accurate abstraction of data from the patient record, interrater agreement was carefully monitored. Each member of the research team who participated in data collection was trained by the project director and had to achieve a 90% agreement on each measurement before independent data were collected. In addition, a detailed rule book was kept so that reliability could be maintained. Interrater reliability was checked on a random selection of 10% of records and maintained at 90% agreement between coders. Whenever agreement dropped below 90%, differences in scoring were analyzed and resolved, usually through the construction of additional coding rules.

Cost. Two sources of financial information were used in this study: charge data from actual patient bills and cost data from the hospital's cost management information system (CMIS). The CMIS uses product- or service-specific cost data provided by each hospital department. In most cases, the costs per product or per service delivered were derived by calculating the actual cost of material and labor, such as a CAT scan or physical therapy session, projecting the estimated volume of all services, and then adding a weighted portion of that department's indirect cost to each product or service. Room costs included only direct cost of nursing salaries, including benefits, and unit specific costs such as equipment depreciation and supplies. While questions of accuracy always arise, the method of calculating specific costs at the level of individual products or services delivered is generally acceptable and is as close to "true" costs as possible at this setting. A variety of analyses were performed on these data and a fuller description is provided in another publication (Douglas, Daly, Rudy, Song, & Dyer, in press). The comparisons between DRG weight, total charges for the entire hospitalization, total costs, total payment or reimbursement from any payor, the margin, study period charges, and charges and costs to produce a survivor are described in this report.

DRG weight is the adjustment for variance of complexity used by the federal government for diagnosis-related groups. The margin is the difference between the cost of each patient's care and the reimbursement or payment actually received. Charges accruing after the patient entered the study were also obtained by subtracting the prestudy period charges from the total hospitalization charges. The cost and charge to produce a survivor in each of the study environments was also calculated by adding the charges (or costs) for every study patient in each unit and then dividing this total by the number of survivors in that unit.

■ Results

The results are presented according to each patient outcome that was compared (see Table 2). When data were in interval level, ANOVA was used with significance set at p ≤ .05. When nominal level data were compared, a chi-square statistic was used with significance set at p ≤ .05.

Mortality: Although a higher percentage of patients cared for in the ICUs died in the hospital (41.3% versus 30.3% for the SCU), this difference was not statistically significant. While a higher percentage of patients from the SCU were discharged home (n = 45; 31%) or to a rehabilitation facility (n = 21; 14.5%), these differences were also not significant.

Length of Stay: The hospital length of stay (LOS) for the total sample ranged from 8 to 176 days, with an overall mean of 49.3 days. There was a large standard deviation in both groups of patients. While the mean LOS for the SCU patients was 2 days less than the ICU patients, this difference was not significant.

Readmission: A total of 17 patients were readmitted to the hospital after discharge. The SCU percentage at 8% is significantly (p = ≤ .03) lower than the ICU's at 20%.

Infections: The total number of infections ranged from 0 to 10 for both groups with an overall mean of 1.6 (SD = 2.3) and with no difference between the groups. Approximately one-third of the patients in both groups had respiratory infections and one-third had urinary track infections. Only 9% (n = 13) of the SCU patients had sepsis (blood infections) compared to 16% (n = 12) of ICU patients. None of the differences noted between the groups was significant.

Respiratory Complications: In both groups, the number of respiratory complications ranged from 0 to 7, with an overall mean of 2.17 (SD = 1.9) per patient and with no significant difference between groups. Only 1% (n = 2) of SCU patients had adult respiratory distress syndrome (ARDS) versus 5% (n = 4) of ICU patients.

Life-Threatening Complications: There was no difference between the groups in the number of life-threatening complications, with an average of about one life-threatening complication per patient. However, the SCU patients had significantly more documented episodes of bradycardia (pulse < 40 BPM), 14.5% vs. 3% in the ICUs (p ≤ .006), and more episodes of a decrease in neurological status (SCU 13% vs. ICUs 4%, p ≤ .033).

Table 2. Comparison of Patient Outcomes Between ICU Patients and SCU Patients[a]

Variable	Special Care Unit $n = 145$	Intensive Care Unit $n = 75$	Stat	p Value	Effect Size	Power
Mortality			$\chi^2 = .66$	.103	.05	.36
Died	44 (30.3%)	31 (41.3%)				
Lived	101 (69.7%)	44 (58.7%)				
Discharge disposition from hospital:			$\chi^2 = 4.55$	.473	.14	.33
Died	44 (30.3%)	31 (41.3%)				
Other hospital	3 (2.1%)	0 (0%)				
Long-term care	31 (21.4%)	14 (18.7%)				
Rehabilitation	21 (14.5%)	11 (14.7%)				
Home	45 (31.0%)	19 (25.3%)				
Home ventilator	1 (0.7%)	0				
Length of hospital stay (days)	48.6 ± 29.5 (9 to 160)	50.6 ± 33.4 (8 to 176)	$F = 0.20$	.655	.03	.07
Readmit[b]			$\chi^2 = 4.65$	.031	.18	.48
Yes	8 (8%)	9 (20%)				
No	93 (92%)	35 (80%)				
Total number of infections	1.6 ± 2.3 (0 to 10)	1.7 ± 2.3 (0 to 10)	$F = 0.27$	.870	.02	.05
Total number of respiratory complications	2.14 ± 1.9 (0 to 7)	2.25 ± 1.9 (0 to 7)	$F = 0.10$	.688	.03	.06
Life-threatening complications	1.12 ± 1.4 (0 to 8)	.88 ± 1.2 (0 to 5)	$F = 2.16$	.1917	.09	.26

[a]Continuous variables reported as $M \pm SD$, with range noted below.
[b]The n used for this calculation included only patients who survived to discharge ($n = 145$).

Patient and Family Satisfaction: No difference was noted between the groups on either patients or family satisfaction. The overall patient satisfaction scores ranged from 43 to 105 ($M = 90.1$), and the family satisfaction scores ranged from 125 to 210 ($M = 186.5$). Satisfaction scores were all skewed to the high end of the scale with minimal variability for nearly all patients and family members. Because of this, data collection on this variable was discontinued after two years.

Cost: Comparisons of financial data associated with the two study environments are shown in Table 3. Although the differences in total charges, costs, and margin were not significantly different, both charges and costs were lower for patients in the SCU by 6% to 7%. Combined with the lower mortality rate in the SCU, this resulted in both significantly lower costs and charges to produce a survivor. The actual cost savings were $5,000 less per patient in the SCU, and the cost to produce a survivor was $19,000 less in the SCU versus the ICU. SCU charges were also significantly lower when the prestudy period (prior to the point at which the patient became eligible for the study and experimental patients were transferred into the SCU) was excluded.

■ Discussion

While the original expectation of ICUs was for short-term stays during a vulnerable period of an acute illness, patients today may require life-support technology with intensive monitoring and care for extended periods. These chronically critically ill represent a subgroup of patients whose outcomes of care have not been carefully examined and whose care may be equally effective outside the traditional ICU setting.

The similarity in outcomes is striking considering the differences in the two environments. The special care unit environment was purposely planned to have less technology, be more open to visitors, have less ambient noise and distraction through the use of private rooms, and patient care managed by nurse case managers. The lack of differences between the groups including mortality and length of stay indicate that chronically critically ill patients can be cared for outside the standard ICU setting when their care is managed by skilled nurse case managers. The study confirms that care managed by nurses working with collaboratively derived medical protocols produces outcomes that are equal to or that exceed those of patients whose care is managed by residents and interns in the routine ICU setting. While a significantly lower percentage of SCU patients required readmission, the effect size and power were low, indicating a need for a larger sample size.

The average LOS for all patients was extremely long and therefore costly in terms of intensive care resources. Because of the wide variability in length of stay (8 to 176 days), those patients at the extreme end of the spectrum should be examined. Patients who require intensive care services up to three

Table 3. Comparison of Finance Data Between ICU Patients and SCU Patients[a]

Variable	Special Care Unit $n = 145$	Intensive Care Unit $n = 70$	F	p Value	Effect Size	Power
Charges	$151,226 ± $92,621 (29,388 to 586,139)	$162,718 ± $107,818 (26,621 to 548,829)	.6792	.4107	.05	.12
Payment	$65,709 ± $46,391 (0 to 212,452)	$66,364 ± $55,452 (0 to 305,362)	.0084	.9272	.01	.04
Cost	$76,077 ± $45,101 (13,853 to 231,125)	$81,212 ± $50,186 (9,436 to 251,000)	.5832	.4459	.05	.11
Margin	$−10,899 ± $39,241 (−153,795 to 103,184)	$−14,694 ± $48,083 (−138,015 to 131,297)	.3806	.5379	.04	.09
DRG weight	8,230 ± 5,708 (.451 to 16,986)	8,579 ± 6,039 (.5123 to 16,986)	.1783	.6733	.00	.04
Study period charge	$69,132 ± $53,222 (9,330 to 277,239)	$94,045 ± $85,915 (7,474 to 472,470)	5.3394	.022	.17	.69
Charge per survivor	$215,351 ± $85,303 (98,690 to 482,733)	$279,870 ± $110,407 (139,522 to 661,730)	14.5741	.0002	.30	.95
Cost per survivor[b]	$109,220 ± $45,117 (48,007 to 265,279)	$138,434 ± $44,736 (66,467 to 234,619)	12.684	.0005	.30	.95

[a]Continuous variables reported as $M ± SD$, with range noted below.
[b]The n used for this calculation included only survivors; SCU $n = 101$. ICU $n = 41$.

months are obviously a major financial and personnel burden to hospitals. This calls for an examination of such patients beyond simple mortality statistics to questions of functional status, quality of life, and family response to an extended critical illness. Patients such as the chronically critically ill survive one complication only to develop another. Thoughts regarding the futility of care in some cases of elderly patients with multiple complications, setbacks, and prolonged lengths of stay need to be addressed by the entire health care team before health care providers are forced into making decisions solely on the basis of cost. To provide a fuller picture of the differences between the two groups, post-hoc effect size and power were calculated for each of the fiscal variables (Borenstein & Cohen, 1988; SOLO Power Analysis, 1992). The differences in the fiscal aspects of care associated with the SCU environment were marked. It is important to note that these differences do not represent savings associated only with reduced nursing care or lower nurse-patient ratios. In fact, the nurse-patient ratio for each patient was nearly identical to that found in ICUs, with the exception of the night shift when the ratio in the SCU was occasionally 1:3 rather than 1:2 or 1:1 in the ICUs. Use of cost data, rather than charge data, confirms the conclusion that the differences between the study units was not just a reflection of charging different rates for the SCU.

The primary source of savings in the SCU stems from a different philosophy and approach to the care of these very ill patients. Most ICUs, quite appropriately, are founded on the assumption that the goal of care is to preserve life at all costs. Every precaution is taken to identify and prevent complications; the guideline is to err on the side of aggressive intervention. This approach is appropriate for the typical ICU patient who experiences a very brief and very acute episode of a life-threatening, but survivable illness. It is less appropriate and less effective for chronically critically ill patients whose problems are not short-term, whose illness may not be reversible, and whose course is not improved by the use of therapies, each of which carries with it the possibility of iatrogenic harm. By segregating these patients in the current study, it was possible to change the norms underlying the approach to care, to question what gains were to be made by aggressive pursuit of every abnormal diagnostic test, to reduce the use of daily laboratory testing surveillance, and to tailor care to the specific needs and goals of each patient. This resulted directly in reduced use of X rays, blood tests, and some therapies. The management of the patients in the SCU by expert nurses undoubtedly contributed to the success of this conservative approach to care.

The results of this study demonstrate that carefully selected patients can be cared for outside of the ICU setting under the care of well-trained nurse case managers, with no threat to patient outcomes and with significant cost savings. This finding has major implications for the care of long-term critically ill patients. It would seem prudent for those institutions that have such patients to explore the potential for creating a special care unit with trained nurse case managers.

To replicate these results, it is necessary to recognize the sociotechnical theory that underpins the SCU environment of care (Daly et al., 1991; Happ, 1993), thereby creating a work environment that encompasses both a carefully designed physical space for these patients, as well as an expanded case management role for nurses who work in and contribute to the environment of care. A medical director of the unit who not only understands the medical care of critically ill patients but who supports the collaborative development of treatment protocols and the need for consistency of care provided by case managers is an essential part of the model. Thus, the evidence strongly suggests that the use of a special environment for chronically critically ill patients headed by nurse case managers, as reported in this study, offers health care facilities a viable, cost-effective alternative to traditional ICU units, without sacrificing quality care.   NR

Accepted for publication September 22, 1995.
This study was funded in part by a grant from the National Institute of Nursing Research, Grant number R01-NR02248.

Ellen B. Rudy, PhD, FAAN, is dean and professor, University of Pittsburgh, School of Nursing, Pittsburgh, PA.

Barbara J. Daly, PhD, FAAN, is an assistant professor, Case Western Reserve University, School of Nursing, Cleveland, OH.

Sara Douglas, PhD, RN, is an assistant professor, Case Western Reserve University, School of Nursing, Cleveland, OH.

Hugo D. Montenegro, MD, is an associate professor, School of Medicine, Case Western Reserve University, Cleveland, OH.

Rhayun Song, PhD, RN, was project director during the time of the study at Case Western Reserve University, School of Nursing, Cleveland, OH.

Mary Ann Dyer, MSN, RN, is project staff, Case Western Reserve University, School of Nursing, Cleveland, OH.

▪ References

Ali, J., Serrette, C., Wood, L. D. H., & Anthomisen, N. R. (1985). Effect of postoperative intermittent positive pressure breathing on lung function. *Chest, 85,* 192–196.

American Association for Respiratory Care. (1991). A study of chronic ventilator patients in the hospital. Dallas: Author.

Bartlett, J. G., O'Keefe, P., Tally, F. P., Louie, T. J., & Gorbach, S. L. (1986). Bacteriology of hospital-acquired pneumonia. *Archives of Internal Medicine, 146,* 868–871.

Bekes, C., Fleming, J., & Scott, W. E. (1988). Reimbursement for intensive care services under diagnosis-related groups. *Critical Care Medicine, 16,* 470–481.

Berenson, R. A. (1984). Intensive care units: Clinical outcomes, costs, and decision making. Health Technology Case Study 28 (OTA-28). Office of Technology Assessment. Washington DC: U.S. Government Printing Office.

Borenstein & Cohen, J. (1988). Statistical power analysis: A computer program. New Jersey: Lawrence Erlbaum.

Borlase, B. C., Baxter, J. T., Benotti, P. N., Stone, M., Wood, E., Forse, R. A., Blackburn, G. L., & Steele, G. Jr. (1991). Surgical intensive care unit resource use in a specialty referral hospital: I. Predictors of early death and cost implications. *Surgery, 109,* 687–693.

Byrick, R. J., Mindorff, C., McKee, L., & Mudge, B. (1980). Cost-effectiveness of intensive care for respiratory failure patients. *Critical Care Medicine, 8,* 332–337.

Cohen, I. L., Bari, N., Strosberg, M. A., Weinberg, P. F., Waskswan, R. M., Millstein, B. H., & Fein, I. A. (1991). Reduction of duration and cost of mechanical ventilation in an intensive care unit by use of a ventilatory management team. *Critical Care Medicine, 19,* 1278–1281.

Cohen, I. L., Lambrinos, J., & Fein, I. A. (1993). Mechanical Ventilation for the elderly patient in intensive care. Incremented changes and benefits. *JAMA,* 269f–1029.

Cullen, D. J., Civetta, J. M., Briggs, B. A., & Ferrara, L. C. (1974). Therapeutic intervention scoring system: A method for quantitative comparison of patient care. *Critical Care Medicine, 2,* 57–62.

Daly, B. J., Rudy, E. R., Thompson, K. S., & Happ, M. B. (1991). Development of a special care unit for chronically critically ill patients. *Heart and Lung, 20,* 45–51.

Douglas, S., Daly, B., Rudy, E., Song, R., & Dyer, M. A. (in press). Cost effectiveness of a special care unit to care for the chronically critically ill. *Journal of Nursing Administration.*

Efron, B. (1971). Forcing a sequential experiment to be balanced. *Biometrika, 58,* 403–417.

Elpern, E. H., Silver, M. R., Rosen, R. L., & Bone, R. C. (1991). The non-invasive respiratory care unit. Patterns of use and financial implications. *Chest,* 990–208.

Garner, J. S., & Favero, M. S. (1986). CDC guidelines for handwashing and hospital environmental control, 1985. *Infection Control, 7,* 231–243.

Gundlach, C. A., & Faulkner, T. P. (1991). Charge and reimbursement analysis for intensive care unit patients in a large tertiary teaching hospital. *DICP, 25,* 1231–1235.

Happ, M. B. (1993). Sociotechnical system's theory: Analysis and application for nursing administration (tables/charts). *Journal of Nursing Administration,* 23–54.

Hjelm-Karlsson, K. (1991). Using the biased coin design for randomization in health care research. *Western Journal of Nursing Research, 13,* 284–288.

Kappstein, I., Schulgen, G., Beyer, U., Geiger, K., Schumacher, M., & Daschner, F. D. (1992). Prolongation of hospital stay and extra costs due to ventilator-associated pneumonia in an intensive care unit. *European Journal of Clinical Microbiology and Infectious Diseases, 11,* 504–508.

Keene, A. R., & Cullen, D. J. (1983). Therapeutic intervention scoring system: Update, 1983, *Critical Care medicine, 11,* 1–4.

Kirilloff, L. H., Owens, G. R., Rogers, R. M., & Mazzocco, M. C. (1985). Does chest physical therapy work: A review. *Chest, 88,* 436–444.

Knaus, W. A., Draper, E. A., Wagner, D. P., & Zimmerman, J. E. (1986). An evaluation of outcome from intensive care in major medical centers. *Annals of Internal Medicine, 104,* 410–418.

LaMonica, E. L., Oberst, M. T., Madea, A. R., & Wolf, R. M. (1986). Development of a patient satisfaction scale. *Research in Nursing and Health, 9,* 43–50.

Madoff, R. D., Sharpe, S. M., Fath, J. J., Simons, R. L., & Cerra, F. B. (1985) Prolonged surgical intensive care. *Archives of Surgery, 120,* 698–702.

Meinert, C. L., & Tonasicia, S. (1986). *Clinical trials, design, conduct and analysis.* New York: Oxford University Press, pp. 90–112.

Morran, C. G., Finlay, I. G., Mathieson, M., McKay, A. J., Wilson, N., & McArdle, C. S. (1983). Randomized controlled trial of physiotherapy for postoperative pulmonary complications. *British Journal of Anesthesia, 55,* 1113–1116.

Parkhurst, S. M., Blaser, M. J., Laxson, L., & Wang, W. (1985). Surveillance for the detection of nosocomial infections and the potential for nosocomial outbreaks: Development of a laboratory-based system, part 2. *American Journal of Infection Control, 13*(1), 7–15.

Pasmore, W. (1988). *Designing effective organizations: The sociotechnical system perspective.* New York: John Wiley.

Pasmore, W., & Sherwood, J. (1978). *Sociotechnical systems: A source-book.* San Diego, CA: University Associates, Inc.

Risser, N. (1975). Development of an instrument to measure patient satisfaction with nurses and nursing care in primary care settings. *Nursing Research, 24,* 45–52.

Roberts, D. E., Bell, D. D., Ostryzniuk, T., Dobson, K., Oppenheimer, L., Marten, D., Honcharik, N., Cramp; H., Loewen, E., Bodnar, S., Guenther, A., Pronger, L., Roberts, E., & McEwen, T. (1993). Eliminating needless testing in intensive care—an information-based team management approach. *Critical Care Medicine, 21,* 1452–1458.

Rudy, E. B., Vaska, P., Daly, B., Happ, M. B., & Shiao, P. (1993). Permuted block design for randomization in a nursing clinical trial. *Nursing Research, 42,* 287–289.

Schapira, D. V., Studnicki, J., Bradham, D. D., Wolff, P., & Jarrett, A. (1993). Intensive care, survival, and expanse of treating critically ill cancer patients. *Journal of the American Medical Association, 269,* 783–786.

Schwartz, S., & Cullen, D. J. (1981). How many intensive care beds does your hospital need? *Critical Care Medicine, 9,* 625–639.

SOLO Power Analysis (1992). Los Angeles, CA: BMDP Statistical Software.

Teres, D., Rapaport, J., Lemeshow, S., Haber, R., Gage, R. W., & Avrunin, J. S. (1988). Using a severity of illness measurement with critically ill patients to explain cost validity within diagnostic-related groups (abstract). *Critical Care Medicine, 16,* 406.

Wagner, D. P., Knaus, W. A., & Draper, E. A. (1983). Statistical validation of a severity of illness measure . . . Acute physiology score of APACHE. *American Journal of Public Health, 73,* 878–884.

Zimmerman, J. E., Shortell, S. M., Knaus, W. A., Rousseau, D. M., Wagner, D. P., Gilles, R. R., Draper, E. A., & Devers, K. (1993). Value and cost of teaching hospitals: A prospective, multicenter, inception cohort study. *Critical Care Medicine, 21,* 1432–1442.

Family Members' Experiences Living with Members with Depression

Terry A. Badger

Using interview data from 11 family members and grounded theory methods, this study describes family members' experiences in living with a member with depression. Findings suggest that this process can be described as family transformations. In the first stage of this process—acknowledging the strangers within—family members described observing the metamorphosis of the person and other family members, finding socially acceptable explanations, living two lives, searching for reasons and solutions, and hoping for what was. In the second stage—fighting the battle—family members alternated between the strategies of holding their ground (protective) and of moving forward (coercive) to counteract the metamorphosis, and the strategy of working the system to get help for their ill member. In the third and final stage, family members described gaining a new perspective and identified preserving oneself, refocusing on others, redesigning the relationship, and becoming hopeful as strategies used in this stage.

Depression is a public health problem affecting approximately 25 million Americans and their families. The prevalence estimates for lifetime major depression is 17.1%; there is a higher prevalence for women, young adults, and people with less than a college education (Blazer, Kessler, McGonagle, & Swartz, 1994). Most people suffering from depression live with their families, usually their spouses and children. Recent studies of families with members with depression[2] have focused more on the biological causes and treatment of depression and less on its interpersonal context (Beach, Sandeen, & O'Leary, 1990; Coyne, 1990; Keitner, Miller, & Ryan, 1993). Yet the interpersonal nature of depression suggests families have a critical role in both understanding and treating depression.

Western Journal of Nursing Research (1996) 18, 149–171.

The majority of recent studies of families with members with depression have used primarily inpatient samples, have focused on depressed women as the identified patient, have been from the patient perspective, have often excluded parents of children with depression, and are quantitative in methodology (Keitner, Miller, Epstein, & Bishop, 1990; Schwab, Stephenson, & Ice, 1993). This study extends previous work by including the perspectives of seven women whose husbands were depressed, two men whose wives were depressed, and two parents whose children were depressed. The purpose of this study was to describe family members' experiences in living with a member with depression.

■ Related Literature

Families with members with depression experience difficulties with communication, marital adjustment and dissatisfaction, expressed emotion, problem solving, and family functioning (Biglan, Hops, Sherman, Freidman, et al., 1985; Keitner, Miller, Epstein, Bishop, & Fruzzetti, 1987; Schwab et al., 1993). Communication between members with depression and their spouses is characterized by high levels of tension, negative expressions, self-preoccupation, and diminished nonverbal patterns of support. The strain of the poor communication in the couples' relationships often continues after recovery. Couples that include one partner with depression consistently rate higher than control couples on marital difficulties and dissatisfaction (Beach, Sandeen, & O'Leary, et al., 1990).

Although the cause-and-effect relationships of expressed emotion remain unclear, expressed emotion has been found to be significantly associated with increased symptom levels and relapse (Hooley, Orley, & Teasdale, 1986). People with depression are more likely to be criticized by their spouses than other family members. Couples with greater spousal criticism have shown consistently higher relapse rates than control couples (Beach et al., 1990). Further, divorce rates for these couples have been reported as nine times higher than the national average.

It should not be surprising that depression has its most negative impact on families during acute depressive episodes. Negative symptoms such as a lack of interest in social life, fatigue, constant worrying, irritability, and hopelessness were the most disturbing aspects of living with ill family members and caused greater disruption in family functioning and greater burden for family members than did other symptoms (Coyne, Kessler, Tal, Turnbull, et al., 1987; Fadden, Bebbington, & Kuipers, 1987; Miller et al., 1992). In their studies of families with members with depression, Keitner et al. (1990) found that these families showed greater impairment in family functioning than families who contained members with alcohol dependence, adjustment disorders, schizophrenia, or bipolar disorders.

Fortunately, negative symptoms decrease in the approximately 75% of people with depression who respond to treatment (Depression Guideline Panel, 1993). However, studies have consistently found that families with a member with depression continue to experience more difficulties at remission than matched control families. These families continue to experience problems with social functioning one year after initial treatment (Billings & Moos, 1985). Families with remitted members failed to reach the level of social resources (friends, supportive family interactions) observed for control families. Similarly, Keitner et al. (1987) found that 46% of their clinical families reported impairment in their overall functioning at remission in contrast to only 18% of control families.

Families with members with depression report greater health problems than families with other types of illness (Hinrichsen, Hernandez, & Pollack, 1992; Pruchno, Kleban, Michaels, & Dempsey, 1990; Wells et al., 1989). Coyne et al. (1987) found that over 40% of adults living with family members with depressive episodes were distressed themselves to the point of needing therapeutic intervention. The detrimental effect on children living with a parent with depression has also been well documented (Buckwalter, Kerfoot, & Stolley, 1988; Merikangas, Weissman, & Prusoff, 1990). Children of parents with depression exhibit greater symptomatology and impairment than control children, and their risk of developing an affective disorder has been reported as high as 45%. Billings and Moss (1985) had similar findings. The children of parents with depression were still functioning more poorly than control group children one year after remission of parental illness.

■ Method

SAMPLE

Purposeful sampling was used to recruit 11 English-speaking family members who were living or who had recently lived with someone with depression. A combination of advertising at a local mental health clinic and network/snowball sampling in which initial informants referred others to the study was used. Of the family members, 9 were women and 10 were white. A total of 7 family members were wives of men with depression, 2 were husbands of women with depression, and 2 were parents of children (1 son, 1 daughter) with depression. The mean age of the family members was 46 years (ranging from 32 to 61 years). Of the family members, 8 were married, and the mean number of years married was 18:8. A total of 8 had at least a baccalaureate education, and annual incomes ranged from below the poverty level to above $50,000. All people who are termed *members with depression* in this study met standard diagnostic criteria as determined by a psychiatrist or psychologist (American Psychiatric Association, 1994). Members with depression included those currently in acute episodes, in recovery, and at remission.

Although half had been hospitalized, not one was hospitalized at the time of the interview.

DATA COLLECTION

After screening to ensure family members met study criteria, consent forms were signed. Open-ended interviews were usually conducted in the researcher's office because most family members preferred the office over the home setting. These audiotaped interviews lasted between 1 and 2 hours. The following broad data-generating question was used to begin the interview: "Tell me what it has been like living with your [husband, wife, child] who [is/was] depressed." Informants responded with full descriptions to this question, and few subsequent probes or clarifiers were required.

DATA ANALYSIS

Interviews were conducted simultaneously with data analysis (Chenitz & Swanson, 1986; Glaser, 1978; Hutchinson, 1986). Interviews were professionally transcribed and checked by the researcher for accuracy. Each interview was coded and guided the selection of subsequent informants. Open coding was used for the initial analysis of the transcribed data, and initial categories were adjusted with subsequent interviews. Categories were refined by merging categories into smaller sets of higher level concepts to fit the emerging theory. Concurrent coding and analysis continued until unique categories no longer appeared in the data, and no additional informants were obtained after data saturation (Glaser & Strauss, 1967). Verification of the categories occurred as similar patterns from previous interviews appeared over time. A central or core category that best explained the process of living with a person with depression was identified as *family transformations*.

Lincoln and Guba (1985) suggested that four factors can be used to assess the rigor of the qualitative study: credibility, transferability, dependability, and confirmability. Credibility refers to having confidence in the truth of the findings. Methods used to check credibility included peer debriefing, exposure of the investigator's thinking to consultants with expertise in both grounded theory and family members' experiences of living with members with other chronic illnesses, discussion with clinicians who work with people with depression and their families, and member checks with some family members who were asked to verify the emerging constructions. Transferability is concerned with providing sufficient data to enable others to make judgments about the degree of similarity between contexts. The sample included adult family members who provided thick descriptions from their perspectives as husbands, wives, parents, and so forth. Dependability refers to the stability and tracking of the data over time. The researcher used a systematic data management system to track the data by hand using detailed memos. Equivalence checks were also conducted within the interviews by asking similar questions and evaluating consistency of the informants' answers (Brink, 1991). Confirmability was supported by gathering information from a variety of sources, and alternative explanations were explored with both family members and professionals. Colleagues experienced in grounded theory methods functioned as inquiry auditors. Transcribed consultations with these colleagues were used to reexamine, recode, or recategorize portions of the data. Further, initial codings, comparative memos, and process and personal notes were reevaluated, enabling changes in earlier data formulations.

■ Findings

The basic social psychological process of family transformations was identified from the data (see Figure 1). The process refers to the cognitive and behavioral changes that occur within the family from the time the member begins to exhibit symptoms of depression through recovery and at remission. As family members move through the three stages of family transformations, all family members are transformed, and family functioning is changed.

STAGE 1: ACKNOWLEDGING THE STRANGERS WITHIN

Acknowledging the strangers within was described as the stage when family members first acknowledged the profound changes in the member with depression, other family members, and family functioning. Family members

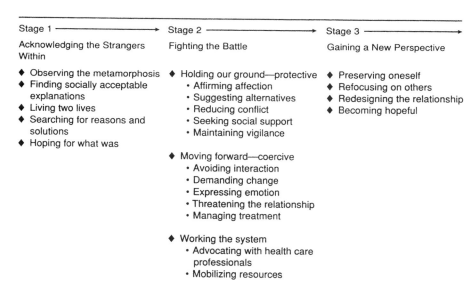

FIGURE 1. Family transformations: stages of living with a member with depression.

described *observing the metamorphosis, finding socially acceptable explanations, living two lives, searching for reasons and solutions,* and *hoping for what was.* The length of this stage varied among family members from months to years, and for some, it was primarily a retrospective process occurring after intervention by a third party.

Family members described observing the metamorphosis of the member with depression. Family members described their member with depression as becoming a completely different person, but they did not associate the metamorphosis with a diagnosis of depression until much later. The following examples illustrate the metamorphosis of the member with depression:[3]

> You are not living with the same person that you've known all these years. He used to be a very patient, very easy-going, very kind, caring person. He's not anybody I recognize at this point. He is very testy, he is very tense . . . there is no hope. (Ida)

> I think the biggest thing for [me], was hard for me to deal with because of my personality and with her, like that she'd be negative. It would just be, and I know it wasn't her and that would make me more angry. (Eddie)

> It's like day and night, Jekyll and Hyde, he's this totally different person. But I see glimmers of him in there . . . it's so discouraging. (Fran)

The depressive symptoms made it difficult, if not impossible, for the members with depression to enact their respective roles and caused difficulties in all areas of family functioning, including communication, problem solving, and marital satisfaction. Other family members, usually the spouse, assumed the role tasks of the ill member. The family atmosphere was described as tense or conflicted, and family members experienced guilt, anger, frustration, and pain. Spouses complained about the lack of emotional or material support from the members with depression and their frustrations with poor parenting:

> What about me? When will he be well enough to give anything back again? . . . when will he be supportive back? (Ida)

> He's been a good provider and we've been married for [many] years. He's been out of a job since last August, and he seems to be unable to hunt for one in a very productive manner. I feel some resentment because the fact that that was always his role. He was always the dependable breadwinner and now he isn't. (Cathy)

> It's frustrating to me to see him and to see his kids. Yeah, when he gets home and there seems to be not much there. And time is going by, . . . and they're still young enough to be excited to see him. And there is going to be a time when all they're going to remember is, he was never around, or he was always tired, or he . . . (Ginger)

The parents of children with depression expressed similar feelings and sentiments: "my stomach would literally churn 'til she got out of bed" (Amy). Although frustrated with the child's behavior, separating from the child was not an option exercised by the parents, unlike spouses who considered separation.

A consistent theme for all family members was the simultaneous metamorphosis of others within the family and the increased physical and mental health problems of family members.

> I never had any experience with depression growing up . . . everyone I knew including me was ok, so I didn't have any experience to draw on. . . . One counselor I went to said I had situational depression . . . I get all emotional but I'm working on it. . . . I think my trust is shot, and that [there are] all the other feelings of rejection and abandonment [crying—unable to continue] . . . I'm sort of a basket case. (Fran)

Several family members had been treated for depression, and others were sufficiently distressed to require counseling. Approximately one-third of the family members reported that their children were affected by living with a parent with depression to the degree that they were beginning to display behaviors similar to the depressed parent. Family members were concerned about their children's genetic vulnerability to developing depression as well as the effect of the current social environment:

> My fear right now though is that my daughter has, is depressed. I don't know enough about this yet, but she is so much like her Dad. And the older she is getting, the more I see it . . . if this is hereditary . . . if children can have it, then I want to do something that will help her. . . . I don't know if I should be removing the children from it or not. Because I think they are sheltered from it because he is [either working or sleeping], but I'll probably find out in 10 years, they'll come back . . . and go "you know, Mom . . ." (Ginger)

Children within the family expressed the loss of parental love and attention. One loss was due to the illness, and the other to the well parent's caring for the ill member. One daughter expressed their sentiments: "Although I didn't want to be sick like Dad, but in a way if I was, I would get all the attention" (Ida). Parental family members expressed that these comments supported leaving the marriage to avoid exposing the children to the parental depression.

Finding socially acceptable explanations was used to explain the metamorphosis and to protect against potential stigma. Reasons that would be considered rational explanations to the average person were used to explain the changes: relationship losses, job stresses, marital difficulties, other illnesses, or personal behaviors of other family members. Explanations, particularly those perceived as having little stigma attached to them, were usually suggested:

> Her mother died. . . . And [the change] was very, very dramatic. And understandable, . . . I shared in her grief, . . . I fully expected, as a normal person would, . . . to deal with the grief, and recover. . . . These were my expectations and that didn't occur. She did change, but she was not the same socially, sexually, or intellectually. (Ben)

> And at first we attributed it to his back pain and not that it was depression, but that his change and attitude change and personality change and response toward the children was all because of his pain and not really related to any depression. To this day even though he will admit he is severely depressed, it is seen as a tremendous sign of weakness. (Ida)

Almost all family members at one time questioned their responsibility in causing the behavior. Family members attributed particularly the irritability and anger to be caused by their own behavior:

> I would say in the last year that I even realized that that is what the problem was. . . . For a long time I thought it was me. If I did something, if I did it differently, if I reacted differently, . . . I thought, well, he's an alcoholic, and that's the problem . . . he's a workaholic and that's the problem or . . . (Ginger)

Unfortunately, finding socially acceptable explanations could prolong suffering because it interfered with or prevented the accurate recognition and treatment of depression.

Living two lives was used to maintain the illusion to the outside world that all was well within the family. This strategy also defended against potential embarrassment or stigma:

> In the beginning, I told no one. I guess I felt embarrassed and didn't want to admit that my son had problems, that he had [attempted suicide]. That was so hard, to come to work and act like all was well, with my friends too. (Hazel)

> I was living two lives, trying to live the life in the house, trying to survive in the house and raise two children, and then trying to maintain a job, and save face here, and never letting anyone know what was going on. That was real hard. (Diane)

> Now with his friends, it's been horrible, because I have to lie to them, I have to be evasive . . . [they ask] what is going on? . . . I [say] everything's fine, we've just been really busy with . . . (Karen)

Family members told no one about the problem, isolated themselves from others, and exhibited stoicism by suppressing painful feelings or selectively sharing them within the family home. While they were living two lives, family members expressed profound feelings of aloneness and additional stress from dealing with the members of the extended family. One family member stated, "my mother doesn't want to know when [she] is not doing well, it gets her too upset . . . so I just say, 'oh, [she's] all right' [when asked]" (Amy).

The member with depression was also living two lives. The ill member may have been able to maintain predepression behavior for limited amounts of time, often having just enough energy to function at work or for short periods outside the family home:

> I see him some days and wonder, How can you go to work and maintain? How can you make it? He says, "I smile a lot and I hide in my office a lot" . . . I don't know how he can do it . . . so I guess there is some strength there. (Fran)

Thus some family members believed the depressive symptoms and behavior could be controlled. This perception caused family members to express anger and hurt about what was perceived as unwillingness by the member with depression to control the behavior.

> He was irritable and unhappy, he would get angry, break things, stayed in his room and listened to [music]. . . . He became terrible at home. . . . The minute he left the house he could turn it off and click, he was fine. He would be all smiles and talkative as if nothing was wrong. . . . He could be yelling and angry and get on the phone to his friends and be fine. Same old [person]. (Hazel)

Until reaching a crisis, finding socially acceptable explanations and living two lives were used sometimes for years. For some, a suicide attempt moved family members quickly into a crisis and toward seeking help for their ill member. Prior to the attempt, these family members were similar to other family members in using the strategies of finding socially acceptable explanations and living two lives. Others described this point as "spinning out of control" (Amy) or "being in a downward spiral with no end in sight" (Jenny). At the point when the family could no longer continue functioning, the family began searching for reasons and solutions to explain the metamorphosis.

Searching for reasons and solutions involved gathering information from both professional and lay literature, and requesting assistance from health care professionals (HCPs), usually the primary care physician. For some family members, their search was often serendipitous. They read about depression in popular magazines or heard about it on television. Interviews with famous people with depression were cited as important resources. One found information at her physician's office:

> We were in a doctor's office one time, . . . and there was a pamphlet on depression and he read it while I was in with the doctor. And when I came out it was like this light bulb went on. After I had been talking to him about this for probably 9 months . . . but he was reading it for himself and for some reason something connected . . . [he] wanted to look

> into it. And so we saw [the doctor] and asked about clinical depression. And he said, "Oh yeah, that's the real thing." (Ginger)

Unfortunately, many HCPs also used the strategy of finding socially acceptable explanations, resulting in misdiagnosis, ineffective treatment, or both:

> And this first [HCP] said that "you're not depressed, you are sad, there's something else other than depression that's wrong with you," and sent him on his merry way. So you know, obviously nothing happened, he wasn't getting any better. So then he decided to [find someone else]. (Fran)

> We got her into a couple of different kinds of therapies. I got her into [alcohol treatment] 'cause we thought alcohol was the problem . . . and when that didn't work we got her into extended care . . . and when that didn't work she saw a private psychiatrist. (Amy)

Family members expressed their frustrations with the health care and insurance systems during this stage. They described seeking help outside their current health care and insurance systems because they were so desperate for help for their ill family member:

> I couldn't tell you how many agencies I tried to get help from. We would go and have one visit and they'd say they couldn't see us anymore. I think if somebody would have sat down and told me what to do, that's really what I wanted. I wanted somebody to say, "This is what's wrong with her, this is what you need to do," and I would have done it. (Amy)

Throughout this first stage and by searching for reasons and solutions, family members experienced hoping for what was. Hoping contained feelings of grief about what was lost and hope for what might be again. As one family member stated, "We had a fairly good relationship . . . so I'm dangling the carrot out here, saying remember how it was" (Ben). Another stated, "we had a wonderful life and I would love to just grasp hold just for a little bit of that" (Karen). Optimism about possible solutions increased the sense that the member with depression and the entire family would return to normal.

STAGE 2: FIGHTING THE BATTLE

Fighting the battle was described as the family members' daily efforts to deal with the interactional patterns within the family developed during the first stage that were perceived as different from predepression interactional patterns. These patterns were perceived as destructive to all aspects of family functioning such as communication or problem solving:

> We won't discuss it, we won't fight about it, we won't communicate in any way, shape or form about it. . . . So, not that I want to fight about it, I want to communicate about it and see my way through it. And I feel I don't want to just abandon her, because I know she's there, somewhere, this wonderful person, . . . but I don't know how to get in touch with her. (Ben)

> Probably for our family unit this has been tremendously destructive. . . . I feel it's kinda like living in hell . . . there has been no consistency in our lives. (Ida)

Family members alternated between the strategy of *holding our ground—protective* and the strategy of *moving forward—coercive* to deal with the fragile or vulnerable family member. Choices of strategies were determined by the family members' beliefs about which strategy would be most effective to counteract or control the metamorphosis and return the family to normal. Fighting the battle also involved *working the system* to obtain help for their ill family member.

The protective strategies were designed to prevent the situation from worsening and to protect the vulnerable individual from potential psychological and physical harm. The five protective strategies were *affirming affection, suggesting alternatives, reducing conflict, seeking social support,* and *maintaining vigilance.* Affirming affection was designed to assure the members with depression that they were loved and wanted. For example, some family members used frequent words or endearment to remind the members they were valued members of the family. Others reassured their ill family members that family members' feelings had not changed about them despite their illness. Affirming affection was also used to counter negative self-statements about the member's worth: "I've been able to reiterate how much I feel for her, how much worth she has. I've communicated how special I think she is" (Ben).

A second strategy—suggesting alternatives—involved providing the member with depression with ideas about how to increase pleasurable activities and to decrease depression. These included encouraging the member with depression to engage in hobbies, spend time with family and friends, exercise, return to school, and decrease work time. Family members expended considerable energy in suggesting alternatives. Most family members reported feeling frustrated and angry after using this strategy for any length of time. As family members became increasingly frustrated by their lack of success, they began to decrease communication with the ill family member:

> So I mentioned to him, "Why don't you do something you'll enjoy? Why don't you start trading in [art]?" And he says, "Oh, I couldn't do that." He's, he's just, every positive suggestion that flows from me seems to be met with a negative from him. And because of that, I get tired of even talking to him. (Cathy)

All family members reported using reducing-conflict strategies. These were designed to decrease the potential for conflict or tension within the family. Most often, reducing-conflict strategies were targeted at the negative affectively laden interactional patterns. Strategies included telling the members with depression what the family members believed they wanted to hear, withholding any actually or potentially upsetting news, and refraining from expressing emotion or criticizing the member with depression about expected role behaviors. For example, one woman assumed the task of family finances to avoid any potentially upsetting news or arguments about money. Another stated she no longer asked her husband to do any task because "It's a big deal . . . it's as if he can't cope really with anything" (Ida)

An integral part of reducing conflict was not expressing emotion. This was particularly used when the member with depression initiated conflict by name-calling or using verbal threats. One woman described leaving the house when her husband initiated conflict, but this strategy became increasingly ineffective over time:

> There was a time period that I was leaving the house so much that it was affecting what I was getting done in my own life. I didn't have any clean clothes to wear because I had to leave the house constantly. (Jenny)

Reducing conflict was difficult for other family members, especially children, who perceived that the member with depression was being difficult, angry, or unpleasant without the usual consequences. The most extreme method of reducing conflict was leaving the relationship.

A fourth strategy—seeking social support—was described as family members' attempt to mobilize the social network to maintain their health and well-being. Family members told only those within their social circle who they perceived would be supportive and understanding or who would be nondiscriminatory. All family members reported lacking energy for the typical reciprocity needed to sustain social relationships. They needed friends who could tolerate their lack of reciprocity and who would focus on subjects other than the ill member: "I live it, I don't need to talk about it." (Jenny)

Maintaining vigilance, the final protective strategy, was designed to protect the member with depression from potential self-harm and relapse. It contained elements of uncertainty about whether the vulnerable member would recover. Vigilance behaviors included changing family members' schedules to spend more time with the member with depression, checking on the member's physical and psychological safety, and monitoring progress in taking medication and other treatments. For most family members, maintaining vigilance was an effective method of protecting the vulnerable member during the acute episodes. Maintaining vigilance became counterproductive at remission, causing increased conflict. One woman stated that after her husband expressed suicidal ideation, she changed her work schedule to come home at frequent intervals to monitor him and to constantly check on his medication and other treatments. She continued these vigilance behaviors after her husband was better because of fears of relapse, causing increased conflict in the relationship.

The coercive strategies were also used in fighting the battle. These strategies were designed to force progress and recovery and involved more physical and verbal aggression than protective strategies. They also were described using controlling, tension-inducing, and rejecting terms. These strategies increased when family members became tired or frustrated by the ill member's lack of improvement; when the member with depression had dropped in and out of treatment; when protective strategies had failed to change the behavior; or when family members were unfamiliar with protective strategies.

The coercive strategies were *avoiding interaction, demanding change, expressing emotion, threatening the relationship,* and *managing treatment.* The first strategy—avoiding interaction—was described by family members as eliminating or avoiding communication or contact with the member with depression. Family members who used this strategy were frustrated that protective strategies had not worked. The following is one example of the avoiding-interaction strategy: "we lived separate in the house for [many] years" (Diane). Members with depression were excluded from scripted family routines (e.g., mealtimes) or from particular areas within the household (e.g., spousal bedroom). Family members believed ill members would recognize the exclusion, understand the implications, and modify their behavior accordingly.

The strategy of demanding change was designed to force the members with depression to stop exhibiting depressive symptoms, to engage in treatment, or to resume their roles. Demanding change involved verbal and physical aggression. For example, family members used shaming to demand the person behave as the family members believed was proper. Family members might tell the person to "buck up, pull it together and you'll pull out of it" (Ida) or "act like a man." Shaming generally "made it, I think, even worse" (Ida). Other family members used physical aggression as a method to get the person to enact their roles. For example, one parent physically removed her adolescent from bed so the adolescent would get ready for school, and another family member moved all her husband's belongings into the living room to force him to deal with his withdrawal behaviors. Neither was successful in counteracting the metamorphosis.

Closely related to demanding change was the third strategy—expressing emotions. This strategy involved family members freely expressing their anger or frustration using either verbal or physical methods, and it usually caused escalation in an already conflicted family situation. Family members used name-calling or profanity, and several reported abusing inanimate objects, such as slamming doors, to express their emotions.

Threatening the relationship was used by most family members unless the member with depression demonstrated signs of improvement and active involvement in treatment. For some parents, a modification of the strategy of threatening was asking the child to move outside the family home. The majority of family members questioned their abilities to continue in the marital relationships. For some, actually leaving was seen as a method to force the members with depression to care for themselves and to engage in treatment: "Because it seems to me that as long as I'm there to blame and to be angry at that he may not make any progress. . . . And so in a way, I feel like I'll be doing him a favor" (Cathy)

Managing treatment involved balancing issues of control and responsibility. For some family members, managing treatment was fueled by family members' fears of relapse because they perceived the member with depression as unwilling to engage in or unable to take responsibility for treatment. Others whose members had experienced relapses used this strategy more than other coercive strategies. As family members attempted to manage treatment, issues about control and responsibility surfaced that may or may not have been previous sources of conflict within the relationship:

> [He] was being really noncompliant with his appointments, and as far as medication refills, he hadn't really gotten them. And so then I was really more insistent on trying to make sure he went for help because once I realized that that was truly what it was, then I knew he really needed help. . . . I was driving myself crazy trying to make sure he did go somewheres and get some kind of help and I had to balance that with him not thinking I was being too controlling. (Ida)

Family members alternately engaged in protective and coercive strategies to deal with the interactional patterns between themselves and their ill members. As the ill member engaged in treatment and as depressive symptoms decreased, family members who remained in Stage 2 continued to alternate between these strategies, often regardless of strategy success.

Family members engaged in working the system to obtain help for their ill members. Working the system involved two strategies: *advocating with HCPs* and *mobilizing resources:* Family members advocated to obtain proper diagnosis and appropriate treatment:

> I've had to fight every inch of the way. And it's been a battle, not just with [my husband], but with the people that I would have thought would have been there to support me as far as the care that he needed . . . and I truly believe that if, and I've said this over and over again to [him], if it was a terminal illness, if it was cancer, MS [multiple sclerosis], anything else, the treatment would have been better. It would have been much better, more caring, more concern. And family members would have been more involved and more included. (Ida)

They also assisted their ill members with access, quality, and cost issues related to treatment. Family members mobilized resources. Often, they went outside their current health care and insurance systems and paid for care out-of-pocket. Although described as an economic hardship, all described this as necessary to obtain effective help for their ill members:

> And then even our insurance we found out they won't cover it. I don't know what the counseling or medication is going to cost . . . or whether we're going to be able to afford it. You know, which I really resent that and it makes no sense . . . if the [medication] will help him function normally and make some decent money so he can pay your bill, then you would think they'd want to help him out. (Ginger)

Family members expressed frustration and anger about the care received by the member with depression, the stigma associated with having a mental illness, and their exclusion in treatment.

By the end of Stage 2, family members reported they were physically and emotionally exhausted from fighting the battle. Family members described accepting the realities and limits of their involvement and shifting the focus of responsibility away from the members with depression to others within the family. This was a critical juncture that allowed family members to move into Stage 3:

> At a certain point where I found myself, the shift for me was, a shift of withdrawing emotionally. I started detaching a great deal from the relationship and I lived with him for quite a long time that I wasn't there. I just lost ways of trying to cope with it and I consider myself a very resourceful individual. (Jenny)

> It's really a horrible feeling to know that there is absolutely nothing you can do. If I'm up and happy, it is not going to bring him out of it. (Fran)

> We were talking about it and she told me, very angrily, that it was my fault that she lost her job. And if I hadn't tried to get her outa here, tried to push her to work, she probably would have gone on her own. And something just sorta snapped inside, . . . but it sort of freed me from her. It made me realize that I couldn't fix it. (Amy)

STAGE 3: GAINING A NEW PERSPECTIVE

Gaining a new perspective, the third and final stage, was described as shifting the focus away from the ill member to themselves and others within the family and as changing interactional patterns between family members and the member with depression. As family members moved into Stage 3, they expressed feelings of self-loss and a loss of the person who was. Gaining a new perspective involved *preserving oneself, refocusing on others, redesigning the relationship,* and *becoming hopeful.*

Preserving-oneself strategies were used to regain a sense of self lost while fighting the battle. Other aspects of life such as work, social life, and health practices were changed or put on hold as family members focused on the needs of the ill member. Family members used counseling, setting limits, setting priorities for their own lives, engaging in pleasurable activities, avoiding being around people with depression, and resuming their relationships with others to regain a sense of self:

> When I went back to school I discovered art. And I discovered that I had a love for it, uh, maybe a talent for it and that it was what I wanted to do. It felt right. And I began to feel like I was living my life, that I was really being me. And I became a happy person. I feel like at that point, somewhere along there, I learned how to live and how to live happily. (Cathy)

> I have to know what I want in a relationship, in life. I think that's important . . . good self-knowledge. The best advice I can give [other family members], if they have the capacity to step back and be patient, that's probably the best thing they can do . . . don't allow their lives to start [being] controlled by the other person [with depression]. . . . I don't want to become a victim of her depression. (Ben)

Family members realized that to care for others, they must care for themselves:

> I have to take care of me. I'm important for myself and my family, too. I couldn't live my own life because I was too preoccupied with theirs. I told them. and I said, "I cried a tub full of tears and it never changed a thing." I still care. I care about them, but I cannot live like this, I mean live my life for them completely. That's too much you know. (Diane)

For other family members, self-preservation required separating from or divorcing the member with depression. Those who chose this option expressed tremendous pain associated with the decision but discussed it as a critical step for self-survival and for maintaining their own sanity:

> Yea, that is the sadness part. Because to have that separation due to one person being depressed is a whole different kind of breakup than having a divorce because one partner has gone off and found another partner or whatever. For me, it's not over yet. It's a very definite sensation that I have a legal divorce, but there has not been an emotional divorce, no emotional divorce has occurred. . . . It just finally came down to self-survival. (Jenny)

Within families, refocusing on others involved reestablishing or repairing previous relationships with extended family members and friends. For some family members, it was only at this stage that the extended family was told the truth about the member with depression. For many, it was the first time the metamorphosis was attributed to depression rather than some socially acceptable explanation. Family members described increasing time with their children to counteract the negative effects of living with a parent with depression:

> My daughter has really been flown around in all this too. She doesn't
> know if we're leaving or staying from one day to the next . . . her life cer-
> tainly isn't stable right now and that certainly adds to my pain. I try to re-
> assure her that no matter what happens, . . . she'll never stopped being
> loved no matter where we may live. But I really try to make an effort and
> to leave her out of the day-to-day kind of stuff that I'm going through.
> (Fran)

Family members described redesigning the relationship between the member with depression and other family members as a necessary step to positively reconnecting with the person with depression. Family members learned
to show love, care, and concern for the member with depression while maintaining emotional distance and limiting responsibility. Further, many learned
to enjoy engaging in activities with them or resume living with the members
with depression.

Family members accepted that the old patterns of relating were no longer
productive and may have maintained the depression. Interactional patterns
such as communication or problem solving were examined, and new interactional strategies were developed:

> Just a lot of family dynamics are going to have to change. What specifi-
> cally I'm not sure, but I just think that things will have to be different . . .
> whether it's mental illness or anything two people go through that's this
> overwhelming that you can go back to things being the way they were . . .
> there's no way possible. (Ida)

> Once in awhile she will step back into a negative thing, but rather than ig-
> nore it like before, I tell her. And she'll see it and she'll stop. (Eddie)

> I still realize how it affects us when I talk to him . . . he tries to remind me
> that sometimes he is going to be down, but that doesn't mean he won't be
> all right. I just worry . . . and it has also affected my relationships with
> my daughters as well. (Hazel)

For a few family members, redesigning the relationship occurred through
counseling and family sessions focused on the interactional patterns within
the family. These family members reported more successful outcomes than
family members who did not have such counseling. For some who were unable to redesign the relationship, they separated or divorced.

As part of this third stage, family members described becoming hopeful.
One spouse described her mood following initiation of treatment as follows:
"now I feel like there's hope" (Ida). Another family member stated, "medication helps. . . . I do believe that she's gonna be ok, whatever happens. So I am
optimistic" (Amy). As part of their new perspective, family members accepted
the new realities and limits. Their feelings of hope were mixed with caution,
particularly for those ill members who had relapsed.

■ Discussion

The social psychological process found in this study describes how all family members are transformed when living with members with depression. The grounded theory described the movement of the family members through stages of acknowledging the strangers within, fighting the battle, and gaining a new perspective. The negative symptoms (e.g., hopelessness, irritability) were the most disturbing aspects of the ill member's metamorphosis for many family members, and the metamorphosis of all family members resulted in difficulties in family functioning and health that were sometimes unresolved at remission. These findings support those from previous studies of family functioning and depression. (Coyne et al., 1987; Keitner et al., 1990). Some strategies (e.g., avoiding, threatening) used in fighting the battle were also consistent with previous findings with couples that included one member with depression (Beach et al., 1990).

Aspects of the first stage described in this study were similar to stages experienced by caregivers of Alzheimer's patients and of other chronic illnesses (Hinrichsen et al., 1992; Skaff & Pearlin, 1992; Strauss et al., 1984; Wilson, 1989). For example, there were similarities found for observing the changes in the ill member and others, finding socially acceptable explanations, and hoping for what was. Regardless of the type of illness, family members used rational nonstigmatizing explanations to explain behavioral changes and hoped the person's behavior would return to normal. The stigma associated with depression according to most family members was greater than for other illnesses that have clearer biological bases, such as Alzheimer's. Despite educational efforts to the contrary, mental illness is still associated with moral weakness or failure. The stigma associated with depression often interfered with seeking or continuing in treatment. Family members described sharing the stigma with their member with depression. This phenomenon seems similar to stigma contagion usually associated with deviance research (Kirby & Corzine, 1981). The phenomenon of stigma contagion may explain why family members are often excluded from treatment by members of the health care community. Further, current public policies have made it difficult for families to obtain quality help at reasonable costs for themselves and their ill members.

The sense of self-loss described by family members is similar to that described for Alzheimer's caregivers (Skaff & Pearlin, 1992) and for heart transplantation partners (Mishel & Murdaugh, 1987), among others. As family members focus on the ill member in the initial stages, they assume role tasks previously enacted by the ill member, and they limit social, work, or other roles. Although family members initially believed their lives would eventually return to normal, the reality was that their lives had changed. A critical step for family members to move to the final stage in this and in other studies with other illnesses was accepting the new realities and limiting responsibility for the ill member.

There are some major differences between the illness of depression and other chronic or terminal illnesses. The majority of those with depression will respond favorably to treatment and resume much of their previous functioning. Unlike the typical course of Alzheimer's or AIDS, with progressive decline and eventual death from the illness, most symptoms of depression such as fatigue or poor concentration subside rather quickly following treatment with little or no long-term effects. Although there is a risk of self-inflicted death with depression, the majority of people with depression recover following treatment to live long, productive lives. Death is not the inevitable outcome. The favorable prognosis for depression was a double-edged sword for family members who alternated between hope and frustration while fighting the battle.

This study provides perspectives of family members not normally included in recent depression studies (Coyne, 1990). In contrast to women being the identified patient, most family members in this study were middle-aged women who were the wives and mothers of the members with depression. These perspectives provide a needed dimension for understanding the process of living with members with depression. Process-oriented research expands knowledge about interpersonal and social contexts of depression. Theories addressing the process of living with depression provide an important foundation for understanding and treating depression in families.

Terry A. Badger, Ph.D., R.N., Associate Professor, College of Nursing, University of Arizona, Tucson.

■ Notes

1. The funding for this study was provided by Sigma Theta Tau International, Beta Mu Chapter, Tucson, AZ. The author thanks Drs. Linda Phillips, Alice Longman, and Joan Haase for their consultation throughout this process and comments on earlier drafts of this article. Special thanks to the family members who gave so generously of themselves. An earlier version of this article was presented at the Western Society for Nursing Research Conference in San Diego, CA, in May 1995. Address correspondence to Terry A. Badger, Ph.D., R.N., College of Nursing, University of Arizona, P.O. Box 21023, Tucson, AZ 85721–0203. Electronic mail may be sent to TBadger@RN1.nursing.Arizona.edu.

2. This article will use the more accurate and more cumbersome phrase members with depression instead of depressed members to avoid reducing people to illness labels and to be consistent with the guidelines in the *Diagnostic and Statistical Manual of Mental Disorders* (American Psychiatric Association, 1994).

3. Examples have been slightly edited for clarity and to protect confidentiality. Alterations are noted within the brackets, and authorship using a pseudonym is cited within the parentheses.

■ References

American Psychiatric Association. (1994). *Diagnostic and statistical manual of mental disorders* (4th ed.). Washington, DC: Author.

Beach, S. R. H., Sandeen, E. E., & O'Leary, K. D. (1990). *Depression in marriage: A model for etiology and treatment.* New York: Guildford.

Biglan, A., Hops, H., Sherman, L., Freidman, L. S., Arthur, J., & Osteen, V. (1985). Problem-solving interactions of depressed women and their spouses. *Behavior Therapy, 16,* 431–451.

Billings, A. G., & Moos, R. H. (1985). Psychosocial processes in unipolar depression: Comparing depressed patients with matched community controls. *Journal of Consulting & Clinical Psychology, 53,* 314–325.

Blazer, D. G., Kessler, R. C., McGonagle, K. A., & Swartz, M. S. (1994). The prevalence and distribution of major depression in a national community sample: The National Co-Morbidity Survey. *American Journal of Psychiatry, 151,* 979–986.

Brink, P. J. (1991). Issues of reliability and validity. In J. M. Morse (Ed.), *Qualitative nursing research: A contemporary dialogue* (rev. ed., pp. 164–186). Newbury Park, CA: Sage.

Buckwalter, K. C., Kerfoot, K. M., & Strolley, J. M. (1988). Children of affectively ill parents. *Journal of Psychosocial Nursing and Mental Health Services, 26,* 8–14.

Chenitz, W. C., & Swanson, J. M. (1986). *From practice to grounded theory: Qualitative research in nursing.* Menlo Park, CA: Addison-Wesley.

Coyne, J. C. (1990). The interpersonal processes of depression. In G. I. Keitner (Ed.), *Depression and families: Impact and treatment* (pp. 31–54). Washington, DC: American Psychiatric Press.

Coyne, J. C., Kessler, R. C., Tal, M., Turnbull, J., Wortman, C. B., & Greden, J. (1987). Living with a depressed person. *Journal of Consulting and Clinical Psychology, 55,* 347–352.

Depression Guideline Panel. (1993). *Depression in primary care* (Vols. 1–2, Clinical Practice Guideline No. 5 [AHCPR Publication No. 93–0551]). Washington, DC: U.S. Government Printing Office.

Fadden, G., Bebbington, P., & Kuipers, L. (1987). Caring and its burdens: A study of spouses of depressed patients. *British Journal of Psychiatry, 151,* 660–667.

Glaser, B. G. (1978). *Theoretical sensitivity: Advances in the methodology of grounded theory.* Mill Valley, CA: Sociology Press.

Glaser, B. G., & Strauss, A. L. (1967). *The discovery of grounded theory: Strategies for qualitative research.* New York: Aldine.

Hinrichsen, G. A., Hernandez, N. A., & Pollack, S. (1992). Difficulties and rewards in family care of depressed older adults. *The Gerontologist, 32,* 486–492.

Hooley, J. M., Orley, J., & Teasdale, J. D. (1986). Levels of expressed emotion and relapse in depressed patients. *British Journal of Psychiatry, 126,* 164–176.

Hutchinson, S. (1986). Grounded Theory: The method. In P. L. Munhall & C. J. Oiler (Eds.), *Nursing research: A qualitative perspective* (pp. 116–117). New York: Appleton-Century-Crofts.

Keitner, G. I., Miller, I. W., Epstein, N. B., & Bishop, D. S. (1990). In G. I. Keitner (Ed.), *Depression and families: Impact and treatment* (pp. 3–29). Washington, DC: American Psychiatric Press.

Keitner, G. I., Miller, I. W., Epstein, N. B., Bishop, D. S., & Fruzzetti, A. E. (1987). Family functioning and the course of major depression. *Comprehensive Psychiatry, 1*, 54–64.

Keitner, G. I., Miller, I. W., & Ryan, C. E. (1993). The role of the family in major depressive illness. *Psychiatric Annals, 23*, 500–507.

Kirby, R., & Corzine, J. (1981). The contagion of stigma. *Qualitative Sociology, 4*, 3–20.

Lincoln, Y. S., & Guba, E. G. (1985). *Naturalistic inquiry.* Beverly Hills, CA: Sage.

Merikangas, K. R., Weissman, M. M., & Prusoff, B. A. (1990). Psychopathology in offspring of parents with affective disorders. In G. I. Keitner (Ed.), *Depression and families: Impact and treatment* (pp. 3–29). Washington, DC: American Psychiatric Press.

Miller, I. W., Keitner, G. I., Whisman, M. A., Ryan, C. E., Epstein, N. B., & Bishop, D. S. (1992). Depressed patients with dysfunctional families: Description and course of illness. *Journal of Abnormal Psychology, 101*, 637–646.

Mishel, M. M., & Murdaugh, C. L. (1987). Family adjustment to heart transplantation: Redesigning the dream. *Nursing Research, 36*, 332–338.

Pruchno, R. A., Kleban, M. H. Michaels, J. E., & Dempsey, N. P. (1990). Mental and physical health of caregiving spouses: Development of a causal model. *Journal of Gerontology, 45*, 192–199.

Schwab, J. J., Stephenson, J. J., & Ice, J. F. (1993). Family research in *Evaluating family mental health: History, epidemiology, and treatment issues* (pp. 157–226). New York: Plenum.

Skaff, M. M., & Pearlin, L. I. (1992). Caregiving: Role engulfment and the loss of self. *The Gerontologist, 32*, 656–664.

Strauss, A. L., Corbin, J., Fagerhaugh, S., Glaser, B. G., Maines, D., Suczek, B., & Weiner, C. L. (1984). *Chronic illness and the quality of life* (2nd ed.). St. Louis, MO: C. V. Mosby.

Wells, K. B., Stewart, A., Hays, R. D., Burnam, M. A., Rogers, W., Daniels, M., Berry, S., Greenfield, S., & Ware, J. (1989). The functioning and well-being of depressed patients: Results from the Medical Outcomes Study. *Journal of the American Medical Association, 262*, 914–919.

Wilson, H. S. (1989). Family caregivers: The experience of Alzheimer's disease. *Applied Nursing Research, 2*, 40–45.

Answers to Selected Study Guide Exercises

■ Chapter 1

A. 1.   1. a   2. b   3. c   4. c   5. b   6. a   7. c   8. a   9. c   10. d

A. 2.   1. a   2. b   3. d   4. a   5. b   6. a   7. b   8. d   9. b   10. c   11. a.   12. a

B.   1. Florence Nightingale   2. Nursing education   3. Clinical practice 4. Tradition   5. Inductive   6. Logical positivism (positivism) 7. Determinism   8. Naturalistic   9. Scientific approach   10. Empirical 11. Generalization   12. Reductionist   13. Field   14. Quantitative research   15. Qualitative research   16. Identification

C. 5.   a. Basic   b. Applied   c. Applied   d. Basic   e. Basic f. Applied   g. Basic   h. Applied

■ Chapter 2

A. 1.   1.a   2. c   3. b   4. a   5. b   6. a   7. c   8. c

A. 2.   1. a   2. b   3. c   4. b   5. a   6. a   7. b   8. c   9. a   10. b   11. a   12. b

A. 3.   1. b   2. c   3. b   4. a   5. c   6. c   7. c   8. c

B.   1. Researcher, investigator   2. Subjects, study participants   3. Concepts   4. Variable   5. Categorical   6. Continuous   7. Independent variable   8. Dependent   9. Independent   10. Data   11. Operational definitions   12. Qualitative   13. Patterns of association   14. Cause-and-effect   15. Functional (associative)   16. Qualitative, quantitative 17. Quantitative   18. Research design   19. Sample   20. Empirical (data collection)   21. Data analysis   22. Pilot study   23. Research report 24. Dissemination   25. Gaining entrée   26. Saturation

▪ Chapter 3

A. 1. c 2. d 3. b 4. a 5. c 6. e 7. d 8. b 9. c 10. e 11. b 12. d

B. 1. Oral report, poster session 2. Journal articles 3. Abstract
4. Headings 5. Introduction 6. Method 7. Statistical test 8. Level
of significance 9. Themes 10. Results

▪ Chapter 4

A. 1. d 2. b 3. c 4. b 5. a 6. d 7. b 8. a 9. c 10. a 11. b 12. d

B. 1. Dilemmas 2. Nurenberg code 3. *Belmont Report* 4. Harm
5. Minimal risks 6. Self-determination 7. Full disclosure
8. Anonymity 9. Vulnerable 10. Institutional Review Boards

▪ Chapter 5

A. 1. 1. b 2. c 3. a 4. b 5. a 6. c 7. b 8. a

A. 2. 1. a 2. c 3. d 4. a 5. b 6. d 7. a 8. c 9. b 10. d 11. b
12. c 13. b 14. a 15. c

B. 1. Research problem 2. Research question 3. Research aims, objec-
tives 4. Experience, literature, social issues, theory, external sources
5. Qualitative 6. Introduction 7. Relationship 8. Two
9. Independent, dependent 10. Multivariate, complex
11. Null (statistical)

C. 6

Independent	*Dependent*
4. a. Type of stimulation (tactile versus verbal)	4. a. Physiological arousal
4. b. Nurses versus patients	4. b. Perceived importance of physical versus emotional needs
4. c. Primary versus team nursing	4. c. Patient satisfaction
4. d. Frequency of turning patients	4. d. Incidence of decubitus ulcers
4. e. Patients' gender	4. e. Amount of narcotic analgesics administered
5. a. Prior blood donation versus no prior donation	5. a. Amount of stress

Independent	*Dependent*
5. b. Frequency of initiating conversation	5. b. Patients' ratings of nursing effectiveness
5. c. Nurses' informativeness	5. c. Level of preoperative stress
5. d. Draining versus no draining of peritoneum	5. d. Incidence of infection
5. e. Method of delivery	5. e. Incidence of postpartum depression

▪ Chapter 6

A. 1. d 2. a, b 3. a, b, c 4. a 5. b 6. d 7. a 8. a 9. b, c 10. b, c

B. 1. CINAHL 2. Subject 3. Textword 4. Indexes, abstract journals
5. Primary 6. Research findings 7. Relevance 8. Quotes 9. Gaps
10. Critical summary 11. Tentativeness

▪ Chapter 7

A. 1 1. c 2. e 3. d 4. e 5. d 6. a 7. b 8. d

A. 2 1. c 2. d 3. f 4. a 5. e 6. b

B. 1. Invented (created, constructed) 2. Hypotheses 3. Framework
4. Conceptual models 5. Words 6. Person, environment, health, nursing
7. Induction 8. Health Promotion Model 9. Borrowed theories
10. Grounded

▪ Chapter 8

A. 1 1. b 2. b 3. a 4. d 5. b 6. a 7. d 8. a 9. b 10. d

B. 1. Comparison 2. Independent 3. Treatment (intervention)
4. Systematic bias 5. Random assignment 6. Pretest (baseline measure)
7. Factorial design 8. Levels 9. Double-blind 10. Repeated measure
(crossover) 11. Causality (causal relationships) 12. Comparison
13. Pre-experimental 14. Time series 15. Equal (equivalent) 16. Non-experimental 17. Correlational 18. Independent 19. Causation
20. Retrospective 21. Case-control 22. Longitudinal 23. Follow-up
studies 24. Surveys 25. Evaluation 26. Constancy 27. Protocols
28. Generalizability 29. Internal 30. Selection 31. Maturation
32. History 33. External

C.3.

a. Cannot	b. Can	c. Can	d. Cannot
e. Cannot	f. Cannot	g. Can	h. Cannot
i. Can	j. Can	k. Cannot	l. Can
m. Can	n. Cannot	o. Can	

C. 4.

4. a. Nonexperimental   4. b. Nonexperimental   4. c. Nonexperimental
4. d. Both   4. e. Nonexperimental   5. a. Nonexperimental
5. b. Both   5. c. Nonexperimental   5. d. Both
5. e. Nonexperimental

■ Chapter 9

A. 1.   1. b 2. a 3. d 4. c 5. b 6. a 7. b 8. c 9. d 10. c

A. 2.   1. c 2. a 3. b 4. d 5. a 6. c 7. b 8. c 9. c 10. a

B. 1. Emergent 2. Bricoleurs 3. Anthropology, psychology, sociology
4. Cultures 5. Macroethnography, microethnography 6. Researcher as instrument 7. Essence 8. Spatiality, corporeality, temporality, relationality 9. Grounded theory 10. Constant comparison 11. Complementary 12. Qualitative, quantitative 13. Incremental 14. Validity 15. Instruments 16. Interpretation

C. 2. a. Grounded theory b. Ethnography
      c. Discourse analysis d. Phenomenology

■ Chapter 10

A.1.   1. c 2. a 3. d 4. b 5. c 6. b 7. c 8. d 9. a 10. d

A.2.   1. b 2. c 3. a 4. b 5. b 6. c 7. a 8. a 9. d 10. b

B. 1. Sample 2. Representativeness 3. Biased 4. Homogeneous
5. Accidental sample 6. Strata 7. Judgmental; purposeful; theoretical 8. Simple random sampling 9. Weighting 10. Multistage 11. Sampling interval 12. Sampling error 13. Accessible 14. Increases 15. 30 16. Information 17. Maximum variation 18. Typical case

C. 2 a. Cluster (multi-stage) b. Convenience c. Systematic
       d. Quota   e. Simple random f. Snowball (network)

▪ Chapter 11

A. 1.   1. b 2. a 3. c 4. c 5. d 6. a 7. a 8. c 9. d 10. a

A 2.   1. c 2. b 3. a 4. a 5. c 6. b 7. b 8. a 9. c 10. a

A 3.   1. a,c 2. a,b 3. b,c 4. c 5. b 6. b 7. a,b,c 8. a,b 9. a,b,c 10. a

B. 1. Structure, quantifiability, researcher obtrusiveness, objectivity
2. Historical research   3. Secondary analysis   4. Topic guide   5. Focus group interview   6. Life histories   7. Closed-ended (fixed-alternative)
8. Open-ended   9. Closed-ended (fixed alternative)   10. Scale   11. Declarative   12. Reversed   13. Bipolar adjectives   14. Random   15. Extreme response set   16. Response set biases   17. Vignettes   18. Behavior
19. Reactivity   20. Participant observation   21. Single, multiple, mobile
22. Logs, field notes   23. Category system   24. In vivo   25. In vitro

C. 4. Y = 11; Z = 26

C. 5. A = Acquiescence; B = None; C = Extreme response set; D = Nay-sayers' bias

▪ Chapter 12

A. 1   1. a 2. c 3. b 4. c 5. a 6. b 7. d 8. b

A. 2   1. a 2. c 3. b 4. d 5. a 6. b

B. 1. Attributes (characteristics)   2. Quantification   3. Rules   4. Measurement error   5. True score   6. Stability   7. Cronbach's alpha (coefficient alpha)   8. Interrater (interobserver) reliability   9. Valid   10. Face
11. Content   12. Predictive   13. Construct   14. Psychometric evaluation   15. Credibility, transferability, dependability, confirmability
16. Prolonged engagement   17. Data triangulation   18. Member check
19. Confirmability   20. Inquiry audit

▪ Chapter 13

A. 1.   1. d 2. a 3. d 4. b 5. c 6. a 7. b 8. d 9. c 10. b   11. b 12. a

A. 2.   1. b 2. a 3. c 4. d 5. b 6. b 7. a 8. a 9. c 10. a

A. 3.   1. b 2. a 3. d 4. b 5. c 6. a 7. a 8. a 9. d 10. a

B. 1. Enumeration (count)   2. Ordinal   3. Zero   4. Equal distances
5. Parameter   6. Frequency distribution   7. Frequency polygons
8. Symmetric   9. Negatively   10. Unimodal   11. Normal distribution

(bell-shaped curve)   12. Central tendency   13. Variability   14. Homogeneous   15. Standard deviation   16. Bivariate statistics   17. Negative (inverse)   18. Pearson's *r* (product—moment correlation coefficient)
19. Inferential statistics   20. Normal   21. Type I   22. Parametric
23. Levels of significance   24. Type II   25. *F*-ratio   26. Chi-squared test
27. Multiple regression   28. R   29. .00, 1.00   30. Analysis of covariance   31. Covariate   32. Factor analysis   33. Discriminant function analysis, logistic regression   34. Logistic regression   35. Path analysis, LISREL (linear structual relations analysis)

C.   3. Unimodal, fairly symmetric

C.   4. Mean: 81.8; Median: 83; Mode: 84

C.   7. a. Chi-squared   b. *t*-test   c. Pearson's *r*   d. ANOVA

C.   9. a. Discriminant function analysis or logistic regression
        b. ANCOVA   c. MANOVA   d. Multiple regression

■ Chapter 14

A.   1. a   2. d   3. c   4. a   5. b   6. b

B.   1. Simultaneously   2. Comprehending, synthesizing, theorizing, recontextualizing   3. Indexing, categorizing   4. Constant comparison
5. Open coding   6. Conceptual file   7. Computer programs   8. Themes
9. Quasi-statistics   10. Selective   11. Basic social process   12. Phenomenologic   13. Detailed

■ Chapter 15

A. 1.   1. b   2. c   3. b   4. d   5. b   6. a   7. d   8. c   9. a   10. a
A. 2.   1. b   2. c   3. d   4. b   5. b   6. a   7. c   8. d

B.   1. Accuracy   2. Hypotheses   3. Causation   4. Their data   5. Important (useful)   6. Decisions   7. Strengths, weaknesses (virtues, flaws)
8. Substantive/theoretical   9. Methodologic   10. Ethical   11. Interpretive   12. Stylistic/presentational

▪ Chapter 16

1. c (also d)   2. a   3. b (also a, c, d)   4. d   5. a   6. a (also b, c, and d)
7. c (also a, b, and d)   8. d   9. b (also d)   10. c (also b and d)

B.   1. Research utilization   2. Gap   3. Conduct and Utilization of Research in Nursing (CURN)   4. Replicated   5. Stetler   6. Knowledge-focused, problem-focused   7. Implementation potential   8. Transferability   9. The cost/benefit of not implementing it   10. evaluation

Polit Student Self-Study CD-ROM to A Essentials of Nursing Research: Metho Appraisal, and Utilization, 5E.

This student self-study CD-ROM contains more than 200 NCLE. tions carefully chosen to help you review and study the content **Essentials of Nursing Research: Methods, Appraisal, and Utiliza .. 5E. ..** Study Mode, you receive feedback with rationale for correct and swers following each question. In Test Mode, questions are scored wit.. back available for your review at the conclusion of the test.

SYSTEM REQUIREMENTS:

To run the CD-ROM, your system must meet the following minimum require-ments:

- PC computer with Microsoft 95, Microsoft 98, Windows/NT, or Windows 2000
- Internet Explorer components of the above Windows systems at or above v.4.0
- A 486 with 66 MHz processor (Pentium processor is recommended)
- 12 MB free hard disk space (24 MB during installation)
- 256-color or greater, 800 by 600 pixel resolution graphics capability and monitor
- CD-ROM drive

ADDITIONAL SYSTEM-SPECIFIC REQUIREMENTS:

Windows 95 or Windows 98
- 16MB of RAM minimum (32 MB recommended)

Windows NT Service Pack 4.0 or Windows 2000
- 24 MB of RAM minimum (48 MB recommended)

INSTALLING THE SOFTWARE FROM THE CD-ROM:

1. Insert the CD-ROM into your CD-ROM drive.
2. Click on the Windows Start button, and select Run.
3. At the command line, type "d:\setup.exe" (where d is the letter represent-ing your CD-ROM drive).
4. Click OK.
5. Follow the online instructions to complete installation.

If your computer does not already have Internet Explorer Version 4.0 or higher, the setup program will inform you and do this installation for you. If this hap-pens, when the Internet Explorer installation is complete, repeat the installa-tion procedure beginning at Step 1.

TECHNICAL SUPPORT

If you experience difficulty viewing the text, it may be the result of the color settings on your system. Should you need assistance or you have any ques-tions regarding the use or content of this CD-ROM, please contact our Techni-cal Support department by telephone at **800-638-3030** or **410-528-4532**, by fax at 410-528-4422, or by email at techsupp@LWW.com. Technical Support is available from 8:30 am to 5:00 pm (EST), Monday through Friday.